HEART
BOOK

How to Keep Your Heart Healthy

JEFFREY DACH MD

Heart Book: How to Keep Your Heart Healthy by Jeffrey Dach MD, First Edition.

Copyright 2018 Jeffrey Dach MD All Rights Reserved.
Published by Medical Muse Press

ISBN: 978-1-7324210-0-4 (paperback)

Author Contact information:
Jeffrey Dach, MD
7450 Griffin Road, Suite 180/190
Davie, Florida 33314
Office Telephone 954–792–4663
Website: www.jeffreydachmd.com

Disclaimer: The reader is advised to discuss the information found in these pages with his or her personal physicians and to act only upon the advice of his/her personal physician. This book is not intended as a substitute for the medical advice of a physician. The reader should regularly consult a physician in matters relating to his or her health, particularly in respect to any symptoms that may require diagnosis or medical attention. The authors and the publisher disclaim responsibility for any adverse effects resulting directly or indirectly from the information or advice contained in this book.

Cover by 99Designs.com
Editing by Edward M. Levy edwardlevy.com
Formatting by Deborah Stocco mybookdesigner.com

Introduction

IF YOU ARE WORRIED ABOUT your cholesterol, and the possibility that you might have heart disease, this book is for you. If you already have heart disease, or are taking drugs for your heart, this book is for you. If you have had a cardiac stent or bypass, or are worried about having one, then this book is for you. The good news is that heart disease is reversible, and stenting or bypass is not inevitable. This book will give you the knowledge and tools to monitor, manage, and reverse heart disease, in spite of your mainstream cardiologist.

Be prepared to be shocked and surprised by what you read in this book. Many of the chapters contain material exactly opposite to what you may believe. Do not be daunted in acquiring new information and discarding the old belief systems of the past.

In case you have doubts, allow me to point out this book is heavily referenced to the medical literature. There is a lag time delay of about 20 years for new information to be accepted by mainstream medicine. This book gives you information and tools 20 years ahead of time.

Since I am not a cardiologist, you might ask the obvious question: *What gives me the ability and authority to write a book about coronary-artery disease? Isn't that reserved for the cardiologist?*

Although I am not a cardiologist, I am a board-certified vascular and interventional radiologist. This means I have spent a thirty-year career studying and thinking about atherosclerotic vascular disease (hardening and narrowing of the arteries). The same disease process that occurs in the coronary arteries also occurs in the peripheral vessels. In addition, for the past 15 years I have been working as a clinician, seeing patients in an outpatient clinic. Cholesterol and heart disease are a major concern of every patient I see in the office.

In the chapters that follow, you will be introduced to a useful cardiac test called the calcium score. This is a radiology imaging test using a CT scan (computerized tomography scan), commonly known as at CAT scan. The calcium-score test originated and was first used in radiology. This book empowers you to fully embrace the coronary calcium score, the new game in town and the paradigm shift in management of heart disease.

Thanks and credit for much of this book goes to many others who have contributed so much to the understanding of heart disease:

David Brownstein MD

Matthew J Budoff MD

Thomas Cowan MD

William Davis MD

Edward A. Gill MD

Beatrice Golomb MD

Malcomb Kendrick MD

Thomas E Levy MD JD

Michel de Lorgeril MD

Donald J Miller MD

Harumi Okuyama MD

Paolo Raggi MD

Uffe Ravnskov MD

Rita Redberg, MD

James C. Roberts MD

Stephen Sinatra MD

William R. Ware, PhD

Jonathan Wright MD

Table of Contents

CHAPTER 1 | Cholesterol Mass Hysteria

IF YOU ARE READING THIS book, you are probably concerned about your cholesterol level and risk for heart disease. Maybe your doctor has already given you a statin anti-cholesterol drug for an elevated cholesterol level. Perhaps you already had a stent or cardiac bypass operation, and afterward were given a statin anti-cholesterol drug.

Perhaps you have a high calcium score. This book will give you the good news. Diet and lifestyle modification can slow progression of both athero-sclerotic plaque and your calcium score.

We are all fearful of and obsessed with our cholesterol level. Is it too high, thereby increasing risk for heart attack? Do we have enough of the "good" cholesterol or too much of the "bad" cholesterol? We all believe in the cholesterol theory of heart disease, the idea that high cholesterol causes heart attacks. We all know this must be true, because everybody believes it.

What if our belief in the cholesterol theory of heart disease is a creation of mass-marketing campaigns by the pharmaceutical industry and is not evidence-based medical science. What if our belief in the cholesterol theory of heart disease has been falsified by modern imaging techniques and numer-ous medical studies. What if our belief in the cholesterol theory of heart disease is actually a form of mass hysteria? The goal of this book is to break you out of your spell and empower you to understand, manage, and reverse atherosclerotic heart disease, using diet, lifestyle modification, and the latest imaging tools.

| CHAPTER | Calcium Score, the New Game In Town |
| 2 | |

THE CALCIUM SCORE IS A radiology imaging test which makes an image of the coronary arteries with a CAT scan (Computerized Axial Tomography). The calcium in the artery has higher density than surrounding soft tissues and appears as white with this technique. By placing a cursor over the coronary artery on a computer screen, the amount of calcium can be calculated. The sum of the calcifications in all three coronary vessels equals the total calcium score.

Paradigm Shift

A paradigm shift in the management of heart disease occurred in 2004 with the publication of the Paolo Raggi study on annual calcium-score progression. A less than 15% annual increase in calcium score is associated with a good prognosis, regardless of a high starting calcium score. On the other hand, a greater than 15% annual progression shows poor prognosis, with increasing rate of myocardial infarction (MI). (1)

Cholesterol Levels Were the Same for Both Groups

Although calcium score progression was highly predictive of heart attack, serum cholesterol level was not a useful predictor. There was no difference in LDL cholesterol levels for the 41 heart-attack patients compared to 450 others free of heart attack. **There was no difference!** Dr. Raggi says:

Mean LDL level did not differ between groups (118 mg/dL versus 122 mg/dL, MI versus no MI). (Dr. Raggi 2004) (1)

Dr. Raggi found that LDL cholesterol is a useless marker for predicting future heart attack.

The Patient Is Failing the Statin Drug?

Dr. Raggi's study also showed that, *in spite of statin drug treatment*, 41 of the 500 patients suffered heart attacks over 6 years. These 41 patients had an annual calcium-score progression greater than 15%, in spite of the statin drugs. Annual calcium score progression in the 41 heart-attack patients was 42% compared to 17% for the 454 event-free survivors. (1) This casts considerable doubt on ability of statin drugs to curb the atherosclerotic process and prevent myocardial infarction. Dr. Matthew Budoff, writing in 2017 on annual calcium score progression, says:

> *I want you to think that if someone is on a statin or not and they are progressing (meaning the calcium score is progressing), they are failing their current therapy. (7)*

Why Is Calcium Score a Superior Predictor Over Cholesterol?

Cholesterol level is measured in the blood-stream, distant from the wall of the artery where the atherosclerotic pathology is located. With the calcium score test, we are measuring the pathology (calcification) directly in the wall of the artery. Progression of calcium score indicates progression of pathological change in the wall of the artery. This is why calcium score is a superior predictor of future heart attack compared to serum cholesterol.

Chronic Inflammatory Foci

Dr. Moeen Abedin (2004) discusses this pathological change in the wall of the artery, stating that vascular calcification is a marker for atherosclerosis, the result of chronic inflammation.

> *Vascular calcification is a clinical marker for atherosclerosis and may represent a special example of the general phenomenon of soft tissue calcification surrounding chronic inflammatory foci. (2)*

Soft-tissue calcification in response to infection is well known and is commonly seen with modern imaging techniques in human bacterial, fungal, and parasitic infections. I would propose that the chronic inflammation in the wall of the artery is a response to polymicrobial infection with biofilm formation. Biofilm is a sticky coating composed of micro-organisms embedded in a slimy extra-cellular matrix.

Tuberculous pericarditis is a good example of soft tissue calcification involving the pericardium, the membrane enclosing the heart. In this disease, CAT-scan imaging typically shows a white rim of calcification encasing the heart. (3) This pattern of calcification in the pericardium is curvilinear and visually similar to arterial calcification, which is also curvilinear. The important point is that calcified pericardium is not caused by elevated cholesterol. Why, then, should we believe that elevated cholesterol causes calcification in the wall of an artery? In fact, Dr. Harvey Hecht has found no correlation between cholesterol levels and calcium score, disproving the idea that cholesterol causes coronary artery calcification. (6) As you will read in the following chapters, a much more plausible explanation is that calcification is caused by infection, a fact that has been confirmed, as we will see, by modern 16s ribosome techniques.

Cholesterol and Calcium Score—No Correlation

Dr. Hecht reported in 2001 that there is no correlation between serum cholesterol and the calcium score. (6) This non-correlation proves that cholesterol does not cause calcification in the coronary arteries. In addition, according to Dr. Edward Gill in a 2010 report, five randomized controlled studies show that statin drug treatment (which reduces cholesterol), does not reduce coronary calcium score or slow progression. (5) Worse, the statin treatment showed a progression of coronary calcium score indistinguishable from the non-treated placebo group. (5)

Calcification Caused by Microbial Organisms

In case you have any lingering doubts about the ability of microbes to cause calcification, I suggest you visit the southern coast of England, where you will find the White Cliffs of Dover. Extending 10 miles, the cliffs are composed of the shells of photosynthetic microbes. These calcified shells accumulate as sediment on the ocean floor over thousands of years, and eventually compacted into chalk, calcium carbonate. Yes, it's true. One-celled microbial organisms make tons of calcium.

Leaky Gut and Vascular Infection

If microbial infection is responsible for vascular calcification, the next question is: *Where is the infection coming from? What location in the body is seeding this infection?* The two most common areas for seeding infection are the gut lining (that is, "leaky gut") and periodontal disease. (12–14) This topic is covered in more detail in chapter 14.

The Leaky Gut Epidemic

Leaky gut has increased to epidemic proportions in our population. (15) Leaky gut is a syndrome in which food particles and gram-negative micro-organisms (endotoxins known as LPS) leak through the gut barrier into the bloodstream. The immune system recognizes these food particles and micro-organisms along with their endotoxins as foreign invaders. This triggers an immune response against them. Through the mechanism of "molecular mimicry", the immune system may mistakenly attack our own tissues causing auto-immune disease.

As a result of "leaky gut", gram negative micro-organisms have now gained entry to the bloodstream and may set up house inside the coronary arteries at sites of shear stress injury; at bifurcations (the Y branching where the vessel splits into two vessels); or at places of movement, such as the coronaries embedded on the surface of a beating heart. Leaky gut is commonly caused by wheat gluten sensitivity in susceptible individuals and/or NSAID (Non-Steroidal Anti Inflammatory) Drugs used as pain killers. Glyphosate, a commonly used herbicide, may represent another cause for the "Leaky Gut" epidemic. On a practical level, testing the patient for anti-gliadin antibodies, which indicates an immune response to gluten, as well as testing for anti-LPS antibodies can be useful in confirming the diagnosis of "Leaky Gut".

Mainstream Cardiology in Denial

In 2004, the cholesterol panel was replaced by the calcium score in routine management of heart disease. This is the paradigm shift in management of heart disease. Yet more than a decade later, mainstream cardiology is still in denial, having buried and ignored Dr. Raggi's 2004 study. The financial stakes are just too high to give up on the cholesterol myth and the billions of dollars made from cholesterol drugs.

To paraphrase Upton Sinclair, *"You can't get a cardiologist to understand something when his salary depends on his not understanding it."*

Nevertheless, the paradigm shift has occurred: Coronary artery disease is polymicrobial infected biofilm, seeded from the gut, and best managed with the calcium score. The cholesterol myth is dead.

It's Time to Let the Older Cholesterol Panel "Rest in Peace"

One cardiologist who has made the transition to calcium scoring is Khurram Nasir, MD, MPH, of Baptist Health South Florida, Miami. Dr. Nasir stated in a session of the 2017 annual meeting of the Society of Cardiovascular Computed Tomography:

> It's time that we should let traditional risk scores and risk factor-based management rest in peace..... They have served their "purpose" for the last 50 years and now in 2017, we have the ability to look at the actual disease with calcium testing, which only costs $75 to $100, takes a few minutes, and has a radiation dose almost equivalent to a mammogram. ....CAC (Calcium Score) testing "provides the most precise insight of what your actual risk is so you can tailor the treatment. (7)

◆ ◆ ◆ ◆ ◆

◆ References for Chapter 2

1) Raggi, Paolo, Tracy Q. Callister, and Leslee J. Shaw. "Progression of coronary artery calcium and risk of first myocardial infarction in patients receiving cholesterol-lowering therapy." *Arteriosclerosis, Thrombosis, and Vascular Biology* 24.7 (2004): 1272–1277.

2) Abedin, Moeen, Yin Tintut, and Linda L. Demer. "Vascular calcification: Mechanisms and clinical ramifications." *Arteriosclerosis, Thrombosis, and Vascular Biology* 24.7 (2004): 1161–1170.

3) Goel, Pravin K., and Nagaraja Moorthy. ""Tubercular chronic calcific constrictive pericarditis." *Heart Views*, Winter 2011, 40-41.

4) Ware, William R. "The mainstream hypothesis that LDL cholesterol drives atherosclerosis may have been falsified by non-invasive imaging of coronary artery plaque burden and progression." *Medical Hypotheses* 73.4 (2009): 596–600. cholesterol atherosclerosis falsified coronary artery plaque Ware Medical Hypotheses 2009

5) Gill, Edward A. "Does Statin therapy affect the progression of atherosclerosis measured by a coronary calcium score?" *Current Atherosclerosis Reports* 12.2 (2010): 83–87.

6) Hecht, Harvey S., et al. "Relation of coronary artery calcium identified by electron beam tomography to serum lipoprotein levels and implications for treatment." *American Journal of Cardiology* 87.4 (2001): 406–412.

7) Maxwell, Yael L. "SCCT 2017 coronary calcium scores in 2017: Useful, yes, but hard outcomes data still lacking." Society of Cardiovascular Computed Tomography (SCCT) 2017 Annual Scientific Meeting.

8) Coronary calcium scans: *New York Times* article highlights value and minimizes limitations. Posted by Michael Joyce, a writer-producer with HealthNewsReview. org

9) Grandhi, Gowtham, et al. "Risk reclassification with absence of coronary artery calcium among statin candidates according to American College of Cardiology / American Heart Association (ACC/AHA) Guidelines: Systematic Review and Meta-Analysis." *Journal of the American College of Cardiology* 71.11 (2018): A1675.

12) Kurita-Ochiai, Tomoko, and Masafumi Yamamoto. "Periodontal pathogens and atherosclerosis: Implications of inflammation and oxidative modification of LDL." *BioMed Research International 2014* (2014).

13) Manco, Melania, Lorenza Putignani, and Gian Franco Bottazzo. "Gut microbiota, lipopolysaccharides, and innate immunity in the pathogenesis of obesity and cardiovascular risk." *Endocrine Reviews* 31.6 (2010): 817–844.

14) Vojdani, Aristo. "The role of periodontal disease and other infections in the pathogenesis of atherosclerosis and systemic diseases." *Townsend Letter for Doctors and Patients* (2000): 52–57.

15) Wyatt, Douglas A. "Leaky gut syndrome: A modern epidemic with an ancient solution " *Townsend Letter* 6 (2014): 68–72.

16) Raggi, Paolo. "Natural history and impact of interventions on CAC." *Cardiac CT Imaging*. Springer, Cham, 2016. 121–132.

17) Raggi, Paolo. "Natural history and impact of interventions on coronary calcium." *Cardiac CT Imaging*. Springer, London, 2010. 59–68.

Superiority of Calcium Score Over LDL Cholesterol

RON IS A SEVENTY-TWO-YEAR-OLD RETIRED engineer whose total choles-terol of 174 hasn't changed over the last seven years. This is quite low. Yet, Ron is concerned because his LDL particle number and LDL particle size are "outside the lab range." He is very worried and concerned about his risk for future heart attack. I explained to Ron that the lab range doesn't apply to him. Ron's calcium score is low, his total cholesterol is 174, and he does not have metabolic syndrome (a pre-diabetic state) or diabetes. So, he doesn't need to worry about the LDL particle size or particle number.

What does mainstream cardiology say about the value of LDL particle size and number?

The Quebec Study

This study followed 2072 males over 13 years and found that small dense LDL was associated with increased mortality from cardiovascular disease. (6) So, you might say, *"Wait just a minute here."* It's true, their published chart is very convincing, and the three lines for small dense LDL are nicely separated with greater numbers of small dense LDL associated with increased mortality. (6) However, as pretty as this may look, **correlation is not neces-sarily causation**. If an increased number of small dense LDL particles causes coronary artery disease, then intervention to reduce the small dense LDL particle number should be preventive. Yet a new study shows this is false. Reducing small-particle LDL with a new drug **FAILS** to reduce heart-attack rate compared to placebo!!

New Drug Reduces Small LDL, but Confers No Benefit in Preventing Heart Disease

Treatment with the new cholesterol-lowering drug evacetrapib resulted in significant decreases in *"total LDL particle number (LDL-P) (up to -54%), and small LDL particle (sLDL) (up to -95%) concentrations."* (5) Yet, according to Dr. Michael Lincoff in *New England Journal of Medicine* 2017, *"treatment with evacetrapib did not result in a lower rate of cardiovascular events than placebo among patients with high-risk vascular disease."* (4)

As a matter of fact, Eli Lilly abandoned development of evacetrapib after this failed study. (4) So, we see that reducing total LDL particle number, or increasing LDL particle size did not confer the benefit of preventing death from heart disease. The benefit was the same as it was for a placebo.

Anacetrapib, another CETP inhibitor similar to evacetrapib under development by Merck had a similar outcome. The drug reduced LDL cholesterol and increased high density lipoprotein (HDL) cholesterol yet did not prevent heart attacks. In October 2017, Merck announced it would not seek FDA approval and abandoned its development. (29)

Dr. Janie Allaire agrees that LDL particle size is not very useful. In Current *Opinion in Lipidology* (2017), she writes:

> LDL particle size . . . has not been independently associated with CVD risk after adjustment for other risk factors such as LDL cholesterol, triglycerides, and HDL-C and that routine use of information pertaining to particle size to determine and manage patients' risk is not yet justified. (1)

In other words, according to Dr. Allaire, the LDL particle size is not a good predictor of cardiovascular risk. (1)

Dyslipidemia of Metabolic Syndrome and AODM (Adult Onset Diabetes Mellitus)

We still have yet to explain the association of small dense LDL with increased mortality from cardiovascular disease. The answer is fairly obvious.

Increased small dense LDL particles are a marker for metabolic syndrome and diabetes mellitus (Type 2 diabetes), both of which are associated with accelerated cardiovascular disease. The pattern of "diabetic dyslipidemia," an abnormally high number of lipids in the blood, is described nicely by Dr. Rivas-Urbina:

Diabetic or atherogenic dyslipidemia, is characterized by high levels of triglycerides and apoB, low concentration of high density lipoprotein (HDL) cholesterol, and increased postprandial lipidemia. This abnormal lipid profile is typical of diabetes but it is also present in prediabetic situations such as insulin resistance and metabolic syndrome. . . . This means that at a given LDL cholesterol concentration, diabetic patients have a greater number of LDL particles. (9)

Dyslipidemia with small-particle LDL is merely a marker for metabolic syndrome. Metabolic syndrome and diabetes itself are associated with high risk for accelerated cardiovascular disease. (7–10) As we have seen, the failed drug study with evacetrapib shows that there is no point in modifying lipoprotein subfractions (LDL particle size and number) with a drug while ignoring metabolic syndrome.

The best way to achieve a reduction in cardiovascular risk is to address the underlying metabolic syndrome, with its pattern of overweight, insulin resistance, elevated blood sugar, and elevated Hgb A1c. This is best achieved by diet and lifestyle modification to reduce blood sugar, weight, and blood pressure. Other interventions such as Metformin and Berberine may be useful for blood-sugar control.

Leaky Gut and Low-Level Endotoxemia

Studies show that patients with metabolic syndrome and diabetes have leaky gut with low-level endotoxemia, implicated in the pathogenesis of many diseases. (13) Dr. Robert Munford (2016) states: (11)

Gram-negative bacterial endotoxin (LPS) has been invoked in the pathogenesis of so many diseases—not only as a trigger for septic

shock, once its most cited role, but also as a contributor to athero-
sclerosis, obesity, chronic fatigue, metabolic syndrome, and many other
conditions. (11)

Low-level endotoxemia from leaky gut triggers release of inflammatory cytokines such as IL-6. (13) This inflammatory state is a direct cause of coronary artery disease. (12) Low-Level endotoxemia is associated not only with inflammation but also infection of the arterial wall. Modern testing techniques have shown that atheromatous plaque—a reversible accumulation of debris in the artery wall—is infected biofilm, an infection with polymicrobial micro-organisms. (17–21) In other words, atherosclerotic plaque is infected biofilm. Individuals can address leaky gut with the well-known protocol of a gluten-free diet, probiotics, glutamine, colostrum, berberine, aged garlic, etc. and thereby prevent the progression of their calcium score and the accumulation of plaque.

Predicting Risk: LDL Subfraction vs. Calcium Score

Calcium score correlates closely with mortality from cardiovascular disease and myocardial infarction. People with a calcium score of zero have the best survival rate, while those with a calcium score over 400 have the worst chance of survival. The CAT coronary angiogram with IV contrast injection provides images of the coronary artery lumen similar to conventional coronary angiography done in the cardiac cath lab. Like the conventional angiogram, the CAT angiogram may show areas of stenosis or blockage in the coronary arteries making this test a useful add-on to the calcium score to aid in discrimination. (22)

The next question you might ask is: *If the cholesterol lipoprotein panel is useful only as a marker for metabolic syndrome, and is not useful as a predictor of risk for coronary artery disease, then what better test should we use to predict risk for cardiovascular disease?*

The answer is the calcium score, an inexpensive test that uses a CAT scan to measure the amount of calcium in the coronary arteries. (23) Studies show the higher calcium score, the greater the risk, the lower the score, the less risk for heart attack. (22) None of the cholesterol subfractions can provide this type of information, and should therefore be relegated to the medical museum, as relic of the past.

Serial Calcium Scores Reveal Response to Treatment

A progression of calcium score less than 15% per year implies benign prognosis. However, a progression of calcium score greater than 15% annually indicates a poor prognosis. The most important chart can be found in Figure 5 from Hecht 2015 (25), originally from Raggi 2004(28).

◆　◆　◆　◆　◆

◆ References for Chapter 3

1) Allaire, Janie, et al. "LDL particle number and size and cardiovascular risk: Anything new under the sun?" *Current Opinion in Lipidology* 28.3 (2017): 261–266.

2) Lawler, Patrick R., et al. "Discordance between circulating atherogenic cholesterol mass and lipoprotein particle concentration in relation to future coronary events in women." *Clinical Chemistry* 63.4 (2017): 870–879.

3) Cantey, Eric P., and John T. Wilkins. "Discordance between lipoprotein particle number and cholesterol content: An update." *Current Opinion in Endocrinology, Diabetes and Obesity* 25.2 (2018): 130–136.

4) Lincoff, A. Michael, et al. "Evacetrapib and cardiovascular outcomes in high-risk vascular disease." *New England Journal of Medicine* 376.20 (2017): 1933–1942.

5) Nicholls, Stephen J., G. Ruotolo, H. B. Brewer, et al. "Evacetrapib alone or in combination with statins lowers lipoprotein(a) and total and small LDL particle concentrations in mildly hypercholesterolemic patients. *Journal of Clinical Lipidology* 2016;10:519–527.e4.

6) St-Pierre, Annie C., et al. "Low-density lipoprotein subfractions and the long-term risk of ischemic heart disease in men: Thirteen-year follow-up data from the Quebec Cardiovascular Study." *Arteriosclerosis, Thrombosis, and Vascular Biology* 25.3 (2005): 553–559 and "Low density lipoprotein Risk of ischemic heart disease." *Arteriosclerosis, Thrombosis, and Vascular Biology* 2005

7) Mooradian, Arshag D. "Dyslipidemia in type 2 diabetes mellitus." *Nature Reviews Endocrinology* 5.3 (2009): 150.

8) Schofield, Jonathan D., et al. "Diabetes dyslipidemia." *Diabetes Therapy* 7.2 (2016): 203–219.

9) Rivas-Urbina, Andrea, et al. "Modified low-density lipoproteins as biomarkers in diabetes and metabolic syndrome." *Frontiers in bioscience* (Landmark edition) 23 (2018): 1220–1240.

10) Sánchez-Quesada, José Luis, and Antonio Pérez. "Modified lipoproteins as biomarkers of cardiovascular risk in diabetes mellitus." *Endocrinología y Nutrición* (English Edition) 60.9 (2013): 518–528. Lipoproteins as biomarkers of cardiovascular risk diabetes mellitus Sánchez Quesada *Endocrinología Nutrición* 2013

11) Munford, Robert S. "Endotoxemia—menace, marker, or mistake?." Journal of leukocyte biology 100.4 (2016): 687–698.

12) *Curr Cardiol Rev.* 2016 Sep 1. Endotoxin, Toll-like Receptor-4, and Atherosclerotic Heart Disease. Horseman MA1, Surani S, Bowman JD.

13) Hawkesworth, S., et al. "Evidence for metabolic endotoxemia in obese and diabetic Gambian women." *Nutrition & diabetes* 3.8 (2013): e83.

14) Gomes, Júnia Maria Geraldo, Jorge de Assis Costa, and Rita de Cássia Gonçalves Alfenas. "Metabolic endotoxemia and diabetes mellitus: A systematic review." *Metabolism: Clinical and Experimental* 68 (2017) and *Clinical Andrology* 8 (2017): 133–144.

15) Tremellen, Kelton, Natalie McPhee, and Karma Pearce. "Metabolic endotoxaemia related inflammation is associated with hypogonadism in overweight men." *Basic* 27.1 (2017): 5.

16) Tremellen, Kelton. "Gut endotoxin leading to a decline in gonadal function (GELDING)—A novel theory for the development of late onset hypogonadism in obese men." *Basic and Clinical Andrology* 26.1 (2016): 7.

17) Hansen, Gorm Mørk, et al. "Pseudomonas aeruginosa microcolonies in coronary thrombi from patients with st-segment elevation myocardial infarction." *PLOS One* 11.12 (2016): e0168771.

18) Ziganshina, Elvira E., et al. "Bacterial communities associated with atherosclerotic plaques from Russian individuals with atherosclerosis." *PLOS One* 11.10 (2016): e0164836.

19) Jonsson, Annika Lindskog, et al. "Bacterial profile in human atherosclerotic plaques." *Atherosclerosis* 263 (2017): 177–183.

20) Lanter, Bernard B., Karin Sauer, and David G. Davies. "Bacteria present in carotid arterial plaques are found as biofilm deposits which may contribute to enhanced risk of plaque rupture." *mBio* 5.3 (2014): e01206–14.

21) Allen, Herbert B., et al. "Arteriosclerosis: The novel finding of biofilms and innate immune system activity within the plaques." *Journal of Medical and Surgical Pathology* 1.135 (2016): 2. Arteriosclerosis novel finding of biofilms within the plaques Allen HB J Med Surg Pathol 2016

22) Al-Mallah, Mouaz H., et al. "Does coronary CT angiography improve risk stratification over coronary calcium scoring in symptomatic patients with suspected coronary artery disease? Results from the prospective multicenter international CONFIRM registry." *European Heart Journal–Cardiovascular Imaging* 15.3 (2013): 267–274.

23) New Zealand Society of Cardiology Position Statement on Coronary Calcium Score (2017).

24) Davis, William. "How to reduce coronary calcium Score." Nov 2017 Wheat Belly Blog.

25) Hecht, Harvey S. "Coronary artery calcium scanning: Past, present, and future." *JACC: Cardiovascular Imaging* 8.5 (2015): 579–596.

26) Demasi, Maryanne, Robert H. Lustig, and A. Malhotra. "The cholesterol and calorie hypotheses are both dead—it is time to focus on the real culprit: Insulin resistance." *Pharmaceutical Journal* doi 10 (2017).

27) Niedzwiecki, Aleksandra, and Matthias Rath. "Nutritional supplement program halts progression of early coronary atherosclerosis documented by ultrafast computed tomography." *Journal of Applied Nutrition* 48 (1996): 68–78.

28) Raggi, Paolo, Tracy Q. Callister, and Leslee J. Shaw. "Progression of coronary artery calcium and risk of first myocardial infarction in patients receiving cholesterol-lowering therapy." *Arteriosclerosis, Thrombosis, and Vascular Biology* 24.7 (2004): 1272–1277.

29) Anacetrapib failure marks the death of the CETP class of cholesterol-lowering therapies. Global Data Healthcare (October 2017) www.drugdevelopment-technology.com/comment/anacetrapib-failure-marks-death-cetp-class-cholesterol-lowering-therapies.

Statin Denialism: An Internet Cult with Deadly Consequences

AN EDITORIAL BY CLEVELAND CLINIC cardiologist Steven Nissen, MD, in the *Annals of Internal Medicine* lamented the problem of **"statin denialism"** on the Internet. (1–2) Dr. Nissen's editorial reveals that the Mom and Pop bloggers operating out of their basements have convinced millions of American to stop taking their statin drugs. Dr Nissen considers this a problem.

They Are Not the "Real Problem"

I propose that Mom and Pop bloggers are not the real problem. The real problem is the "statin drug denialist" residing in the halls of academic medicine. These are the University medical professors who publish their "statin denialism" articles in the mainstream medical literature. One "statin denialist" in the academic cardiology community is Dr. Edward A. Gill, Professor of Cardiology at the University of Colorado. Dr. Gill has actually **DENIED** that statin drugs have any benefit for reducing calcium score.

I just can't believe that! Dr. Gill states that

five randomized controlled trials have demonstrated that not only does statin treatment not reduce coronary calcium, but in fact, the progression of coronary calcium by CT scanning is indistinguishable from placebo treatment. (3)

Another denialist is William R. Ware, PhD, Emeritus Professor University of Western Ontario Canada, who wrote in 2009 that modern imaging studies have falsified the cholesterol theory of atherosclerosis. Dr. Ware says:

Contrary to the conventional wisdom, total cholesterol (TC) and LDL cholesterol in asymptomatic individuals are not associated with either the extent or progression of coronary plaque, as quantified either by electron beam tomography (EBT) or coronary CT angiography. (4)

Dr. Ware also says this data has been largely ignored by mainstream cardiology:

The evidence falsifying the hypothesis that LDL drives atherosclerosis has been largely ignored. (4)

Autopsy Studies Do Not Correlate

Dr. Ware mentions another "inconvenient truth." A review of multiple autopsy studies shows **no correlation** between degree of coronary atherosclerosis and serum cholesterol levels. (18–20)

Statins Stimulate Atherosclerosis and Heart Failure

Another statin denialist is Professor of Biochemistry Harumi Okuyama of Nagoya City University, Japan, who published his 2015 article in the *Expert Review of Clinical Pharmacology*. (22) Dr. Okuyama states that statin drugs actually *stimulate* rather than prevent atherosclerosis. Statins act as toxins to deplete ATP (the molecule responsible for intracellular energy transfer), which is why people on statins may have muscle weakness and muscle pain. Statins also inhibit the synthesis of vitamin K2, which protects arteries from calcification, and seleno-proteins, which protect against congestive heart failure. Dr. Okuyama writes:

Statins may be causative in coronary artery calcification. Statins are mitochondrial toxins that impair muscle function through the depletion of Coenzyme Q10 and "heme A," and thereby ATP generation. Statins inhibit synthesis of vitamin K2, cofactor for matrix Gla-protein activation, which protects arteries from calcification. Statins inhibit biosynthesis of seleno-proteins, a factor in congestive heart failure, reminiscent of the dilated cardiomyopathies seen with selenium deficiency. The epidemic of heart failure and atherosclerosis may paradoxically be aggravated by the use of statin drugs. (22)

Pharmacological evidence and clinical trial results support the interpretation that statins stimulate atherogenesis by suppressing vitamin K2 synthesis and thereby enhancing artery calcification. Statins cause heart failure by depleting the myocardium of CoQ 10, "heme A" and selenoproteins, thereby impairing mitochondrial ATP production. In summary, statins are not only ineffective in preventing CHD (coronary heart disease) events but instead are capable of increasing CHD (coronary heart disease) and heart failure. (22)

Another statin denialist is Dr. Mikael Rabaeus, a cardiologist in Geneva, Switzerland. He writes (2017) that statin discontinuation could actually **SAVE LIVES**!

Statin discontinuation does not lead to increased IHD (Ischemic Heart Disease) and overall mortality.... On the contrary, one might even conclude that statin discontinuation could save lives. . . In summary, it cannot be considered as evidence based to continue to claim that statin discontinuation increases mortality or that statin therapy saves lives. (21)

These denialists are not Mom and Pop bloggers on the internet. These statements are in the mainstream medical literature!!!

Heart-Attack Victims Have Low Cholesterol

If cholesterol was truly the cause of heart attacks, then one would expect heart-attack victims to reveal the high cholesterol causing their heart attack. Researchers found the opposite. Heart-attack victims have low cholesterol. A 2009 study by Dr. Amit Sachdeva analyzed 137,000 heart-attack patients from 541 U.S. hospitals and found that their mean cholesterol was only 174. (10) This is low, not high.

Henry Ford Hospital Heart-Attack Victims

In addition, if high cholesterol were truly the cause of heart attacks, one would expect heart-attack victims with the highest cholesterol to have the worst prognosis, and those with the lowest cholesterol to have the best prognosis. They don't. A 2009 study from Henry Ford Hospital in Detroit showed that three years after a heart attack, the patients with lowest cholesterol had the highest mortality, and those with the highest cholesterol had the best survival **(14% vs. 7%)** (11).

Falsifying the Cholesterol Theory: The Paolo Raggi Study of 2004

As we have seen, the 2004 Paolo Raggi study followed 500 men who were taking statins for coronary artery disease. (23) Calcium scores and cholesterol panels were done annually over 6 years. Forty-one men suffered heart attacks during the 6 years of follow-up. If cholesterol were the cause of heart attacks, then these 41 heart-attack victims should have higher cholesterol than the other 459 heart-attack-free men, and the men who were free from heart attack should have a lower cholesterol that "protected" them. Quite to the contrary, Dr. Paolo Raggi reported the cholesterol levels were the same for both groups, thus disproving the theory that cholesterol causes heart attacks. (23)

The Elderly

A dozen studies show that low cholesterol in the elderly is a marker for increased mortality, not improved survival. (24-29)

Selected Medical Conditions: Lower Cholesterol Increases Mortality

In selected medical conditions such as congestive heart failure, hemodialysis, chronic obstructive pulmonary disease (COPD), and rheumatoid arthritis, higher cholesterol is associated with improved survival and lower cholesterol with increased mortality. (24–29) This paradox is called "reverse epidemiology."

No Mortality Benefit in Primary Prevention Setting

Another statin denialist, Dr. Kausik K. Ray, MD, from Cambridge, wrote in 2010 that men with elevated cholesterol and no history of heart disease had no mortality benefit from taking a statin drug. Dr. Ray says:

> *Data were combined from 11 studies . . . on 65,229 participants followed for approximately 244,000 person-years, during which 2793 deaths occurred. The use of statins in this high-risk primary prevention setting was not associated with a statistically significant reduction in the risk of all-cause mortality. (13)*

Five Statin Drug Studies

Analyzing data from five statin drug studies (4S, WOSCOPS, CARE, TEXCAPS/AFCAPS and LIPID), Peter R Jackson found a 1% *increase* in mortality after 10 years on statin drugs in people with no pre-existing heart disease (primary prevention). (30) Another statin denialist, Rita Redberg, MD, bluntly writes in the *Journal of the American Medical Association (JAMA)* 2012 that healthy men should not take statins. (14)

Who Benefits from Statin Drugs?

Statin drugs were FDA approved based on a small benefit over placebo for middle-aged men with known heart disease. This is called secondary prevention.

Secondary Prevention of Heart Disease in Males

Considering the media and marketing hype over statin drugs, one would think there must be something to it, so let's take a look at the statin drug studies in the best-case scenario—middle-aged men with known heart disease, also known as secondary prevention. This group has proven mortality benefit, and these are the studies submitted for FDA approval for this class of drugs. Let's take a closer look at the data from two of the most representative secondary prevention studies with statin drugs, the 4S (15–16) and the LIPID Studies (17).

4S Trial with Simvastatin in Scandinavia (15,16) – 0.6% per year

Here is a quick recap of the 4S-Trial data. The 4S trial was done on 4444 patients who had known heart disease, randomized to simvastatin or placebo, and followed for 5.5 years. At the end of the follow-up, the researchers reported 182 deaths in the statin drug group (8.2%) and 256 deaths in the placebo group (11.5%). This provided an absolute mortality benefit of 3.3% over 5.5 years, or 0.6% per year. The 6-year probabilities of survival for placebo was 88.5% and for simvastatin was 91.8%, a difference of 3.3%. (15–16)

LIPID Pravastatin Study (17) – 0.5% per year

Here is a quick recap of the LIPID Trial data. Nine thousand patients with unstable angina and a history of myocardial infarction were randomized to either placebo or Pravastatin and followed for 6.1 years. (17)

The statin group had 11% mortality and the placebo group had 14.1% mortality over 6.1 years. This is a 3.1% mortality benefit over 6.1 years or 0.5% per year. After 6 years, probability of survival in the placebo group is 85.9% and 89% in the statin group, a difference of 3.1%. (17)

Absolute Mortality Benefit of 0.5% per year in Secondary Prevention

So, as you can see from the above, the absolute mortality benefit in the best-case scenario, in secondary prevention trials, is only 0.5% – 0.6% per year. This benefit is underwhelming; it is actually quite shocking that it is so minimal, especially since drug-company marketing suggests a much larger benefit.

Perpetuating the Myth

The benefits of statin drugs have been over hyped, and their adverse effects underplayed., You have already met a number of dissenting physicians who have earned the label of "statin denialists" by casting doubts on statin drugs. These "statin denialists" have shown that the benefits of statin drugs are minor, in the range of a 0.5% per year reduction in absolute mortality for middle-aged men with known heart disease. For all other categories, such as women, the elderly and healthy males, there is no benefit, and there are drawbacks relating to the adverse effects of statin drugs. The benefit of statin drugs are related to the anti-inflammatory "pleiotropic effects", rather than any reduction in serum cholesterol. Perpetuation of the statin drug myth is essential for maintaining drug-industry profits. The financial stakes are high, so don't expect change anytime soon.

♦ ♦ ♦ ♦ ♦

♦ References for Chapter 4

1) Nissen, Steven E. "Statin denial: An Internet-driven cult with deadly consequences." *Annals of Internal Medicine.*

2) Husten, Larry. "Cardio brief: Statin denialism is a deadly Internet-driven cult: Steve Nissen says the battle for patients' hearts and minds is being lost." *CardioBrief* July 24, 2017.

3) Gill, Edward A. "Does statin therapy affect the progression of atherosclerosis measured by a coronary calcium score?" *Current Atherosclerosis Reports* 12.2 (2010): 83–87.

4) Ware, William R. "The mainstream hypothesis that LDL cholesterol drives atherosclerosis may have been falsified by non-invasive imaging of coronary artery plaque burden and progression." *Medical hypotheses* 73.4 (2009): 596–600.

5) Steven Nissen conflicts of interest disclosure: Dr. Nissen reports grants from Esperion Therapeutics during the conduct of the study; grants from Amgen, grants from Pfizer, grants from Astra Zeneca, outside the submitted work.

6) Steven Nissen reported receiving research support from Amgen, Abbvie, AstraZeneca, Cerenis, Eli Lilly, Esperion Therapeutics, Novo-Nordisk, The Medicines Company, Orexigen, Pfizer, and Takeda and consulting for a number of pharmaceutical companies without financial compensation (all honoraria, consulting fees, or any other payments from any for-profit entity are paid directly to charity, so neither income nor any tax deduction is received).

7) Sayer, Ji. "Cleveland Clinic Dr. shamelessly promotes statin drugs calling side effects 'imagined.'" July 26th 2017. GreenMedInfo. www.greenmedinfo.com/blog/deadly-internet-driven-cult-drives-statin-denialism-says-clev-clinic-dr.

8) Naughton, Tom. "I admit it: I'm a member of the cult," by Tom Naughton in Bad Science, Media Misinformation, Random Musings.

9) Will Stopping Statins Kill People? The statin skirmishes of recent years have turned into bitter conflict. Dr. Nissen says stopping statins will lead to many deaths. What about side effects? Joe Graedon July 27, 2017 *People's Pharmacy.*

10) Sachdeva, Amit, et al. "Lipid levels in patients hospitalized with coronary artery disease: an analysis of 136,905 hospitalizations in Get With The Guidelines." *American heart journal* 157.1 (2009): 111–117.

11) Al-Mallah, Mouaz H., et al. "Low admission LDL-cholesterol is associated with increased 3-year all-cause mortality in patients with non ST segment elevation myocardial infarction." *Cardiology journal* 16.3 (2009): 227–233.

12) Barakat, Amr F., et al. "Perioperative statin therapy for patients undergoing coronary artery bypass grafting." *The Annals of thoracic surgery* 101.2 (2016): 818–825.

13) Ray KK, Seshasai SR, Erqou S, et al. Statins and all-cause mortality in high-risk primary prevention: a meta-analysis of 11 randomized controlled trials involving 65,229 participants. *Arch Intern Med.* 2010;170(12):1024–1031,

14) Redberg, Rita F., and Mitchell H. Katz. "Healthy men should not take statins." JAMA 307.14 (2012): 1491–1492. Healthy men should not take statins Redberg Rita Mitchell Katz *JAMA* 2012

15) Kjekshus, John, Terje R. Pedersen, and Scandinavian Simvastatin Survival Study Group. "Reducing the risk of coronary events: evidence from the Scandinavian Simvastatin Survival Study (4S)." *The American journal of cardiology* 76.9 (1995): 64C-68C.

16) Pedersen, Terje R., et al. "Lipoprotein changes and reduction in the incidence of major coronary heart disease events in the Scandinavian Simvastatin Survival Study (4S)." *Circulation* 97.15 (1998): 1453–1460.

17) Long-Term Intervention with Pravastatin in Ischaemic Disease (LIPID) Study Group. "Prevention of cardiovascular events and death with pravastatin in patients with coronary heart disease and a broad range of initial cholesterol levels." *New England Journal of Medicine* 339.19 (1998): 1349–1357.

18) Lande K, Sperry W, 1936. Human Atherosclerosis in Relation to the Cholesterol Content of the Blood Serum. *Archives of Pathology.* 22:301–312.

19) Paterson, J. C., Rosemary Armstrong, and E. C. Armstrong. "Serum lipid levels and the severity of coronary and cerebral atherosclerosis in adequately nourished men, 60 to 69 years of age." Circulation 27.2 (1963): 229–236.

20) Mathur, K. S., et al. "Serum cholesterol and atherosclerosis in man." Circulation 23.6 (1961): 847–852.

21) Rabaeus, Mikael, Paul V. Nguyen, and Michel de Lorgeril. "Recent flaws in Evidence Based Medicine: statin effects in primary prevention and consequences of suspending the treatment." Journal of Controversies in Biomedical Research 3.1 (2017): 1–10.

22) Okuyama, Harumi, et al. "Statins stimulate atherosclerosis and heart failure: pharmacological mechanisms." Expert review of clinical pharmacology 8.2 (2015): 189–199.

23) Raggi, Paolo, Tracy Q. Callister, and Leslee J. Shaw. "Progression of coronary artery calcium and risk of first myocardial infarction in patients receiving cholesterol-lowering therapy." Arteriosclerosis, thrombosis, and vascular biology 24.7 (2004): 1272–1277.

24) Horwich, Tamara B., and Gregg C. Fonarow. "Reverse epidemiology beyond dialysis patients: chronic heart failure, geriatrics, rheumatoid arthritis, COPD, and AIDS." Seminars in dialysis. Vol. 20. No. 6. 2007.

25) Ahmadi, Seyed-Foad, et al. "Reverse epidemiology of traditional cardiovascular risk factors in the geriatric population." Journal of the American Medical Directors Association 16.11 (2015): 933–939.

26) Myasoedova, Elena, et al. "Lipid paradox in rheumatoid arthritis: the impact of serum lipid measures and systemic inflammation on the risk of cardiovascular disease." Annals of the rheumatic diseases 70.3 (2011): 482–487.

27) Kalantar-Zadeh, Kamyar, et al. "Reverse epidemiology of conventional cardiovascular risk factors in patients with chronic heart failure." Journal of the American College of Cardiology 43.8 (2004): 1439–1444.

28) Kalantar-Zadeh, Kamyar, et al. "Reverse epidemiology of cardiovascular risk factors in maintenance dialysis patients." Kidney international 63.3 (2003): 793–808.

29) Kalanta-Zadeh, Kamyar. "CARDIOVASCULAR AND SURVIVAL PARADOXES IN DIALYSIS PATIENTS: What Is So Bad about Reverse Epidemiology Anyway?." Seminars in dialysis. Vol. 20. No. 6. Blackwell Publishing Ltd, 2007.

30) Jackson, Peter R., et al. "Statins for primary prevention: at what coronary risk is safety assured?." British journal of clinical pharmacology 52.4 (2001): 439–446.

CHAPTER 5

Cholesterol Levels and Atherosclerosis: Autopsy Studies Show No Correlation

AS WE SAW IN CHAPTER 4, Drs. William Ware and Uffe Ravnskov have both pointed out an inconvenient truth. Autopsy studies dating back to 1936 show cholesterol levels do not correlate with the amount of atherosclerosis. (1) (25) If accepted as true, this would indeed disprove the cholesterol theory of atherosclerotic heart disease.

Drs. K. E. Landé and W. M. Sperry in an autopsy study published in the 1936 *Archives of Pathology*, state:

> *In fresh autopsy material in 123 cases of violent death they compared the serum cholesterol content with the lipid content of the aorta. No relationship was present in any age group. It is concluded that the incidence and severity of atherosclerosis in man is not directly correlated with the blood serum cholesterol content. (2)*

Dr. K. S. Mathur published another autopsy study in 1962 in *Circulation,* writing:

> *Two hundred cases were selected from medicolegal autopsies for a study of the relationship of serum cholesterol to the amount and severity of atherosclerosis in the aorta and the coronary and cerebral arteries . . . No correlation could be observed between the serum cholesterol level and the amount and severity of atherosclerosis in the arteries. (3)*

A more recent study of 51 autopsies by Dr. Braz in the 2007 American Journal of Medical and Biological Research showed *that in patients with severe atherosclerosis blood cholesterol and tri-glyceride levels seem to have little influence on coronary lipid content, indicating that other factors may contribute to arterial lipid deposition and plaque formation. (4)*

Dr. Paterson published two studies in *Circulation* in 1960 and 1963 evaluating "Serum lipid levels and the severity of coronary and cerebral atherosclerosis in adequately nourished men, 60 to 69 years of age." Dr. Paterson writes:

No significant relationships, nor any trend toward such relationships, were found in 18 individual analyses concerning the coronary arteries. Furthermore, the mean serum lipid levels were consistently (but not significantly) higher in persons who did not have demonstrable sequelae [signs] of coronary sclerosis at autopsy than in persons who had sequelae. We conclude from these results that the validity of the "lipid theory" of atherosclerosis remains unproved, as far as the coronary arteries are concerned. (5, 6)

Many others have reported similar findings. (7, 8)

Mainstream Cardiology Has Rejected This Information

Of course, as Dr. William Ware has pointed out, mainstream cardiology has ignored and rejected the results of these and other autopsy studies showing no correlation between serum cholesterol levels and the extent and severity of coronary artery disease. (25) Another inconvenient fact ignored by conventional cardiology is that modern imaging studies with calcium scoring have falsified the cholesterol theory of heart disease. (25)

My Neighbor Bill

Last week, I was having a beer in the backyard with my neighbor, Bill, who is recovering from a triple bypass operation. Bill said:

It was my darn cholesterol that caused it. . . . I'm taking Lipitor (statin drug) and my cholesterol is a lot lower now.

I said, "That's great, Bill." People believe that cholesterol causes heart disease thanks to drug-company television advertising. I didn't have the heart to tell Bill that the theory cholesterol causes heart disease has been disproved by numerous studies. I knew he believed in the cholesterol theory of heart disease, and any information to the contrary would probably have induced a state of shock and disbelief. The benefit from statin drugs is not solely from reduction of LDL cholesterol. Rather, the benefit from statin drugs, if any, arises from their pleotropic effects as anti-inflammatory drugs. (17–18)

Pleiotropic Effects Explain Clinical Benefit of Statins (if Any)

Dr. Narasaraju Kavalipati writes:

Over the years, analyses of several clinical studies, including the landmark HPS and ASCOT-LLA trial, reported findings with statins that were inexplicable with the lipid-lowering mechanism alone. (17)

At the same time, the statin drug reduces serum cholesterol, there is a pleiotropic anti-inflammatory effect that is completely independent of the cholesterol-lowering effect. How much clinical benefit is due to cholesterol-lowering, and how much to pleiotropic effects is a matter of debate. According to Dr. Adam Oesterle in *Circulation Research* (2017):

Statins may exert cardiovascular protective effects that are independent of LDL-cholesterol lowering called pleiotropic effects. . . . .The relative contributions of statin pleiotropy to clinical outcomes, however, remain a matter of debate and are hard to quantify because the degree of isoprenoid inhibition by statins correlates to some extent with the amount of LDL-cholesterol reduction. (18)

All the Benefits of Statin Drugs Are Due to Pleiotrophic Effects

The hypothesis that the benefits of statins are due to their pleiotropic effects is supported by the fact that other lipid-lowering drugs using a different mechanism from statins failed to prevent heart attacks or strokes. (23,24) A perfect example is the new drug, evacetrapib, which inhibits cholesterylester transfer protein (CETP inhibitor). Evacetrapib lowers LDL and increases

HDL cholesterol with a different mechanism from statin drugs, which are HMG- CoA Reductase inhibitors. Quite unexpectedly, evacetrapib failed to prevent heart attacks or strokes in a randomized placebo-controlled trial published in 2017 in the *New England Journal of Medicine*, after which the drug was abandoned. (23,24) The CETP inhibitor drugs lower cholesterol, yet had no clinical benefit for preventing heart attacks or "cardiac events."

Statin Drug Studies Before and After 2005

Dr. Michel de Lorgeril, in two articles from 2015 and 2016, reveals an unpleasant fact. (21,22) Because of the Vioxx Scandal, Congress tightened rules for clinical drug trials in 2005. Statin drug studies before 2005 are of questionable validity but after 2005 are more transparent, more honest, and of greater validity. (21,22) Dr. de Lorgeril writes:

> *In conclusion, this review strongly suggests that statins are not effective for cardiovascular prevention. The studies published before 2005/2006 were probably flawed, and this concerned in particular the safety issue. A complete reassessment is mandatory. Until then, physicians should be aware that the present claims about the efficacy and safety of statins are not evidence based. (21)*

Regarding primary prevention of heart disease by statin drugs in healthy patients with only elevated cholesterol and no known underlying heart disease, Dr. Michel de Lorgeril says that statin drugs have no benefit, and their discontinuation might even save lives. (22)

Summary

Many autopsy studies dating back to 1936 show no correlation between cholesterol level and severity of atherosclerotic disease. The clinical benefit of statin drugs, if any, is entirely due to their pleiotropic effects. Reduction of cholesterol with CETP inhibitor drugs does not prevent heart attacks or strokes. (19–25)

◆　◆　◆　◆　◆

♦ References for Chapter 5

1) Ravnskov, Uffe. "Is atherosclerosis caused by high cholesterol?." QJM 95.6 (2002): 397–403.

2) Landé, K. E., and W. M. Sperry. "Human atherosclerosis in relation to the cholesterol content of the blood serum." Arch. Pathol. 22 (1936): 301–312.

3) Mathur, K. S., et al. "Serum cholesterol and atherosclerosis in man." Circulation 23.6 (1961): 847–852.

4) Braz Jr, D. J., P. S. Gutierrez, and P. L. Da Luz. "Coronary fat content evaluated by morphometry in patients with severe atherosclerosis has no relation with serum lipid levels." Brazilian journal of medical and biological research 40.4 (2007): 467–473.

5) Paterson, J. C., Lucy Dyer, and E. C. Armstrong. "Serum cholesterol levels in human atherosclerosis." Canadian Medical Association Journal 82.1 (1960): 6.

6) Paterson, J. C., Rosemary Armstrong, and E. C. Armstrong. "Serum lipid levels and the severity of coronary and cerebral atherosclerosis in adequately nourished men, 60 to 69 years of age." Circulation 27.2 (1963): 229–236.

7) Cabin, Henry Scott, and William C. Roberts. "Relation of serum total cholesterol and triglyceride levels to the amount and extent of coronary arterial narrowing by atherosclerotic plaque in coronary heart disease: quantitative analysis of 2,037 five mm segments of 160 major epicardial coronary arteries in 40 necropsy patients." The American journal of medicine 73.2 (1982): 227–234.

8) Mendez, Jose, and Tejada, Carlos. "Relationship between serum lipids and aortic atherosclerotic lesions in sudden accidental deaths in Guatemala City." The American journal of clinical nutrition 20.10 (1967): 1113–1117.

9) Solberg, Lars A., and Jack P. Strong. "Risk factors and atherosclerotic lesions. A review of autopsy studies." Arteriosclerosis, Thrombosis, and Vascular Biology 3.3 (1983): 187–198.

10) Nitter-Hauge, Sigurd, and Ivar Enge. "Relation between blood lipid levels and angiographically evaluated obstructions in coronary arteries." British heart journal 35.8 (1973): 791.

11) Johnson, K. M., D. A. Dowe, and J. A. Brink. "Traditional clinical risk assessment tools do not accurately predict coronary atherosclerotic plaque burden: a CT angiography study." AJR. American journal of roentgenology 192.1 (2009): 235

12) Reardon, Michael F., et al. "Lipoprotein predictors of the severity of coronary artery disease in men and women." Circulation 71.5 (1985): 881–888.

13) Romm, Philip A., et al. "Relation of serum lipoprotein cholesterol levels to presence and severity of angiographic coronary artery disease." The American journal of cardiology 67.6 (1991): 479–483.

14) Oalmann, Margaret C., et al. "Community pathology of atherosclerosis and coronary heart disease: post mortem serum cholesterol and extent of coronary atherosclerosis." American journal of epidemiology 113.4 (1981): 396–403..

15) von Birgelen, Clemens, et al. "Relation between progression and regression of atherosclerotic left main coronary artery disease and serum cholesterol levels as assessed with serial long-term (≥ 12 months) follow-up intravascular ultrasound." Circulation 108.22 (2003): 2757–2762.

16) Noakes, T. D. "The 2012 University of Cape Town Faculty of Health Sciences centenary debate: "Cholesterol is not an important risk factor for heart disease, and the current dietary recommendations do more harm than good."" South African Journal of Clinical Nutrition 28.1 (2015): 19–33.

17) Kavalipati, Narasaraju, et al. "Pleiotropic effects of statins." Indian journal of endocrinology and metabolism 19.5 (2015): 554.

18) Oesterle, Adam, Ulrich Laufs, and James K. Liao. "Pleiotropic Effects of Statins on the Cardiovascular System." Circulation Research (2017).

19) DuBroff, Robert, and Michel de Lorgeril. "Cholesterol confusion and statin controversy." World journal of cardiology 7.7 (2015): 404.

20) Okuyama, Harumi, et al. "Statins stimulate atherosclerosis and heart failure: pharmacological mechanisms." Expert review of clinical pharmacology 8.2 (2015): 189–199.

21) de Lorgeril, Michel, and Mikael Rabaeus. "Beyond confusion and controversy, Can we evaluate the real efficacy and safety of cholesterol-lowering with statins?." Journal of Controversies in Biomedical Research 1.1 (2016): 67–92.

22) Rabaeus, Mikael, Paul V. Nguyen, and Michel de Lorgeril. "Recent flaws in Evidence Based Medicine: statin effects in primary prevention and consequences of suspending the treatment." Journal of Controversies in Biomedical Research 3.1 (2017): 1–10.

23) Lincoff, A. Michael, et al. "Evacetrapib and cardiovascular outcomes in high-risk vascular disease." *New England Journal of Medicine* 376.20 (2017): 1933–1942.

24) Dashing Hopes, Study Shows a Cholesterol Drug Had No Effect on Heart Health By GINA KOLATA APRIL 3, 2016 New York Times.

25) Ware, William R. "The mainstream hypothesis that LDL cholesterol drives atherosclerosis may have been falsified by non-invasive imaging of coronary artery plaque burden and progression." Medical hypotheses 73.4 (2009): 596–600.

26) Stehbens, William E. "Coronary heart disease, hypercholesterolemia, and atherosclerosis I. False Premises." Experimental and molecular pathology 70.2 (2001): 103–119.

The Art of the Curbside Cholesterol Consult

IN OUR NEIGHBORHOOD, WE TAKE the garbage cans out to the curb twice a week for pickup. Although we grumble about the extra work, it's a good opportunity to get outside the house and say hello to our neighbors. On one such occasion, I had a curbside consult with my neighbor, Bill Jones.

While wheeling the garbage can around, I said, *"How are you doing, Bill?"* Bill said, *"Not too good,"* and then proceeded to show me the Ace bandage on his arm and two bottles of pills his doctor prescribed for his peripheral neuropathy. Bill was having constant burning pain, tingling, and numbness in the arm and hand, day and night, preventing him from sleeping. The pills were generic Neurontin (gabapentin) a drug marketed for treatment of peripheral neuropathy, and Tramadol, a synthetic opiate pain pill.

Knowing that a cocktail of B vitamins and alpha lipoic acid will frequently clear up and heal a peripheral neuropathy, I asked Bill if he was taking any vitamins. (10) His face lit up and he invited me into his house. We sat in the kitchen and he brought out a sheet of paper listing his medications and vitamins.

At the top of the list was Pravastatin, a drug to reduce cholesterol. When I saw this, I immediately knew what was causing Bill's excruciating burning pain in the arm and hand. It was an obvious case of statin-induced neuropathy. (1) My job had been simplified.

I told Bill the statin drug was causing his peripheral neuropathy, so he should stop the drug immediately. I also gave him a list of vitamins to take:

benfotiamine 150 mg three times a day, B12 methylcobalamin 5000 mcg sublingual tabs twice a day, P-5-P form of B6 50 mg. daily, Alpha Lipoic Acid 50 mg three times a day, Ubiquinone form of CoQ-10 100 mg twice a day. (10)

Adverse Side Effects of Statin Drugs

The drug companies have cleverly planted deceptive articles in the media, proclaiming that statin drugs have no side effects. In reality, statin drugs have horrendous adverse side effects that have been documented in the medical literature for over 30 years. This is the ugly side of statins, and it includes peripheral neuropathy, muscle pain, muscle damage, myopathy, cognitive dysfunction and dementia, autoimmune disease, drug-induced lupus, disturbance of immune function, etc. (5)

No Good Reason to Take a Statin Drug

Bill had no evidence of heart disease, his cholesterol levels were perfectly normal, and he should not be taking a statin drug in the first place. Amazingly, his doctors failed to recognize he had a statin-induced neuropathy, and instead gave Bill a worthless ineffective drug, gabapentin, as treatment for peripheral neuropathy, no more effective than placebo. (13) They also gave him an opiate pain pill Tramadol, which is effective for pain relief; however, the price of taking that drug is narcotics addiction. Prescribing an opiate pain pill for a statin-induced neuropathy is misdiagnosis and mistreatment, a medical error of monumental proportions.

Who Benefits from a Statin Drug?

Medical science is clear that statin drugs reduce cholesterol quite well in men and women of all ages. However, no health benefit is obtained from lowering cholesterol in women, the elderly, or men with no underlying history of heart disease. (8) According to Rita Redberg, MD, in an article in the *Archives of Internal Medicine,* healthy men should not take a statin drug. On the other hand, 30 years of statin medical studies have shown a benefit greater than placebo for middle-aged men with known underlying heart disease. (9)

Although this benefit is not impressive, it is enough to justify prescribing a statin drug to men with known heart disease.

Temptation to Profit

Statin drugs are the most lucrative drugs ever, making more than 100 billion dollars for Pfizer. (2) How did Pfizer make so much money? They put on the scary witch-doctor mask and created fear. The fear is: *"if you don't take my drug, you die."* Of course, this is nonsense, but people are willing to believe nonsense if they are frightened enough.

Creating Fear – Medical Marketing of Statin Drugs

Remember the scary witch-doctor masks on display at the museum, originally intended to induce fear in villagers and motivate them to follow the witch doctor's advice? I often laughed and marveled at how primitive these people were. A modern doctor would never stoop so low as to don a scary mask to induce fear in the patient. How can that be part of any effective medical treatment? Our modern medical system is above that. We are not savages living in mud huts. We are civilized. We have nuclear weapons, and the *New York Times*.

Fear-Tactic Advertising

A Pfizer ad for Lipitor reads, *"Which would you rather have, a choles-terol test or a toe tag?* [the ad image shows a corpse with a toe tag]*"*. This is fear-tactic advertising to convince healthy people to take a drug they don't need. (11–12). This is our modern-day equivalent of the witch-doctor scary mask, fear-tactic advertising to sell drugs to healthy people who don't need them. I guess we are not so lofty as we thought.

My Job as a Physician—Unmasking the Witch Doctors

How does one expose the fear-mongering and propaganda of the drug industry, which turns rational humans into lemmings?

Fifty years ago, when I laughed at the witch doctor mask at the Field Museum, I never could have imagined my job would be to expose the ruse of the witch-doctor mask and try to convince healthy people not to become lemmings jumping off the cliff, clamoring for bad drugs they don't need. Of course, this task would be immensely easier if Congress banned Direct to Consumer (DTC) drug advertising, as most other countries have already done.

Two weeks after stopping the statin drug and starting a new vitamin program as listed above, Bill reports his arm and hand pain are considerably improved, and he is very grateful. (10)

♦   ♦   ♦   ♦   ♦

♦ References for Chapter 6

1) Gaist, D., et al. "Statins and risk of polyneuropathy A case-control study." *Neurology* 58.9 (2002): 1333–1337.

2) Lipitor generated more than $100 billion in revenue for Pfizer since it was approved in 1997. *Crain's New York Business* Dec 28, 2011

3) Phan, T., et al. "Peripheral neuropathy associated with simvastatin." *Journal of Neurology, Neurosurgery & Psychiatry* 58.5 (1995): 625–628.

4) Moosmann, Bernd, and Christian Behl. "Selenoprotein synthesis and side-effects of statins." *The Lancet* 363.9412 (2004): 892–894.

5) Chong, Pang H., et al. "Statin-Associated Peripheral Neuropathy: Review of the Literature." Pharmacotherapy: *The Journal of Human Pharmacology and Drug Therapy* 24.9 (2004): 1194–1203.

6) Two Lassa Witch Doctors. Centers for Disease Control and Prevention's Public Health Image Library (PHIL), with identification number #1322.

8) Getting Off Statin Drug Stories by Jeffrey Dach MD

9) Statin Drugs Revisited by Jeffrey Dach MD

10) Head, K. A. "Peripheral neuropathy: pathogenic mechanisms and alternative therapies." *Alternative medicine review: a journal of clinical therapeutic* 11.4 (2006): 294.

11) Frederick Spohn, MD. Fear tactic advertising. *BCMJ*, Vol. 44, No. 2, March, 2002, page(s) 69 — Letters.

12) Mintzes, Barbara. "For and against: Direct to consumer advertising is medicalising normal human experience." *British Medical Journal* 324.7342 (2002): 908.

13) Hyatt, Joel D., et al. "Diabetic peripheral neuropathic pain: is gabapentin effective?." *American family physician* 84.5 (2011): 480–482.

14) Graveline, Duane. "Adverse Effects of statin drugs: a physician patient's perspective." *J Am Phys Surg* 20 (2015): 7–11.

Statin Drugs and Botanicals: Anti-Inflammatory Effects

FOR THOSE WITH HEART DISEASE requiring a coronary artery bypass graft (CABG), the *New York Times* advises we all take statin drugs, since studies show a 50% reduction in mortality for those who take them after CABG. (1) I was somewhat amazed and perplexed by this, since I had already ridiculed the idea that statin drugs prevent surgical complications. Now I thought I might have to eat my hat and retract my statement.

Pleiotropic Effects

The two studies on this statin drug benefit for cardiac bypass, by Curtis and Barakat, refer to the anti-inflammatory "pleiotropic effects" of statin drugs. (2,3) Cardiac bypass is associated with a massive release of proinflammatory cytokines and an intense systemic inflammatory response. Statin drugs help with all this inflammation by down-regulating Nuclear Factor Kappa Beta (NF-κB), the master controller of the inflammatory response. So, yes, there is a potential benefit for statins as anti-inflammatory agents. Statin drugs block the inflammatory cytokine release in the postoperative patient, thus reducing mortality from the procedure.

Lipophilic statin drugs (those that tend to combine with fats or lipids) such as atorvastatin (Lipitor) and simvastatin (Zocor) seem to work best. Surprisingly, the authors comment that there was no proven reduction in myocardial infarction post cardiac bypass with statin drug use. This was a disappointment. The reduction in mortality was thought to be due to the reduction in systemic inflammatory response. There was another benefit—reduction in episodes of atrial fibrillation. (2,3)

It appears the benefit of statin drugs in this population is not as cholesterol-lowering agents but is due instead to the anti-inflammatory properties of statins. If so, then one might consider other anti-inflammatory interventions that down regulate Nuclear Factor Kappa Beta (NF-kB), the protein complex that is involved in inflammation response. Here is a list of widely available botanicals which exert anti-inflammatory effects by down-regulating Nuclear Factor Kappa Beta (NF-κ B).

Anti-Inflammatory Botanicals

- Curcumin
- Ginger (Zingiber officinale)
- Holy basil (Ocimum)
- Polygonum cuspidatum
- Berberine (Coptis chinensis and barberry, Oregon grape)
- Oregano
- Chinese skullcap (baicalin/ oroxylin A)
- Rosemary

Inflammation Triggered by Nuclear Factor Kappa Beta

Inflammation triggered by nuclear factor kappa beta (NF-κB) is upregulated in many diseases, such as osteoarthritis, viral infections, and cancer, so you would be quite correct to surmise that many of these botanicals are useful for them all. These same botanicals would be useful for reducing joint inflammation associated with cartilage loss in osteoarthritis or rheumatoid arthritis. For example, curcumin alone has been proposed as a new paradigm in the management of osteoarthritis.

Anti-Cancer Studies

Studies of curcumin, berberine, ginger, holy basil, and Chinese skullcap have all shown anti-cancer activity. (12–54) Berberine and curcumin are actually synergistic in anti-cancer activity against breast-cancer cells. (24)

Benefits for Cardiovascular Disease

If atherosclerotic cardiovascular disease is caused by inflammation, as many now believe, this would explain many of the benefits of statin drugs, which are anti-inflammatory. Statins were originally developed as anti-cholesterol drugs, and it was only much later that the anti-inflammatory effects were discovered.

Perhaps anti-inflammatory botanicals or herbal remedies would be more effective than statin drugs, with fewer adverse side effects, for reducing calcium score if combined with aged garlic and vitamin K2. We await these future studies. In the meantime, studies using berberine have shown remarkable benefits in the prevention and treatment of cardiovascular disease. (25–29) Curcumin has been shown effective in retarding atherosclerosis in an ApoE mouse model of atherosclerosis. (55) Chinese skullcap (baicalin) has shown a remarkable ability to prevent cardiovascular disease by lowering the oxidation of low-density lipoproteins, which transport cholesterol around the body. When these lipoproteins become oxidized within the cell walls, they can contribute to atherosclerosis (31–35) Dr. Oh Soon Kim, writing in 2015, said that Chinese skullcap works *"by decreasing the oxidation of LDL and suppressing inflammatory responses in macrophages"* (35).

Anti-Viral Herbal Agents

Chinese skullcap has both anti-viral and anti-inflammatory properties. In his book, Stephen Buhner discusses the great 1918 influenza epidemic, a virulent and deadly viral illness that killed more than 50 million people around the world. The danger of this type of viral illness is related to the viral induced "cytokine storm," a severe inflammatory response that overwhelms and kills the patient. Botanicals like Chinese skullcap are not only potent anti-viral agents, they also turn off an individual's cytokine storm, thereby exerting powerful anti-inflammatory effects. (31)

Conclusion

One might wonder about the outcome of a study funded by the National Institute of Health (NIH) comparing the anti-inflammatory effects of statin drugs to botanical products in diverse conditions such as arthritis, atherosclerosis, and cancer, as well as mortality after coronary bypass graft surgery. Perhaps botanicals would have superior anti-inflammatory effects compared to statin drugs, without the adverse effects of CoQ-10 depletion, vitamin K inhibition, myalgia, neuropathy, diabetes, etc. However, considering the current state of NIH research funding, this study would never be funded. It would never happen. In the meantime, those of us who don't have the luxury of time may wish to incorporate anti-inflammatory botanicals into routine use.

♦   ♦   ♦   ♦   ♦

♦ References for Chapter 7

1) "Having Heart Surgery? Don't Stop Your Statins," by Nicholas Bakalar March 16, 2017 *New York Times.*

2) Curtis, Michael, et al. "Effect of Dose and Timing of Preoperative Statins on Mortality After Coronary Artery Bypass Surgery." *The Annals of Thoracic Surgery* (2017).

3) Barakat, Amr F., et al. "Perioperative statin therapy for patients undergoing coronary artery bypass grafting." *The Annals of thoracic surgery* 101.2 (2016): 818–825.

4–11) deleted

12) Fadus, Matthew C., et al. "Curcumin: An age-old anti-inflammatory and anti-neoplastic agent." *Journal of Traditional and Complementary Medicine* (2016). CurcuminRich Double Strength Theracurmin

13) Wang, Ke, et al. "Curcumin inhibits aerobic glycolysis and induces mitochondrial-mediated apoptosis through hexokinase II in human colorectal cancer cells in vitro." *Anti-cancer drugs* 26.1 (2015): 15–24.

14) Dasiram, Jade Dhananjay, et al. "Curcumin inhibits growth potential by G1 cell cycle arrest and induces apoptosis in p53-mutated COLO 320DM human colon adenocarcinoma cells." *Biomedicine & Pharmacotherapy* 86 (2017): 373–380.

15) Ravindran, Jayaraj, Sahdeo Prasad, and Bharat B. Aggarwal. "Curcumin and cancer cells: how many ways can curry kill tumor cells selectively?." *The AAPS journal* 11.3 (2009): 495–510.

16) Shanmugam, Muthu K., et al. "The multifaceted role of curcumin in cancer prevention and treatment." *Molecules* 20.2 (2015): 2728–2769.

17) Zhang, Jianbin, et al. "Curcumin targets the TFEB-lysosome pathway for induction of autophagy." *Oncotarget* 7.46 (2016): 75659–75671.

18) Ansari, Jamal Akhtar, et al. "Anticancer and Antioxidant activity of Zingiber officinale Roscoe rhizome." (2016).

19) Choudhury, Diptiman, et al. "Aqueous extract of ginger shows antiproliferative activity through disruption of microtubule network of cancer cells." Food and chemical toxicology 48.10 (2010): 2872–2880.

20) Manaharan, Thamilvaani, et al. "Purified essential oil from Ocimum sanctum Linn. triggers the apoptotic mechanism in human breast cancer cells." Pharmacognosy magazine 12.Suppl 3 (2016): S327.

21) Manaharan, Thamilvaani, et al. "Antimetastatic and Anti-Inflammatory Potentials of Essential Oil from Edible Ocimum sanctum Leaves." The Scientific World Journal 2014 (2014).

22) Green Tea for Prevention of Skin cancer

23) Peng, W., et al. "Botany, phytochemistry, pharmacology, and potential application of Polygonum cuspidatum Sieb. et Zucc.: a review." Journal of ethnopharmacology 148.3 (2013): 729–745.

24) Wang, Kai, et al. "Synergistic chemopreventive effects of curcumin and berberine on human breast cancer cells through induction of apoptosis and autophagic cell death." Scientific reports 6 (2016).

24a) Sun, Yiyi, et al. "A systematic review of the anticancer properties of berberine, a natural product from Chinese herbs." Anti-cancer drugs 20.9 (2009): 757–769.

25) Zhang, Ming, et al. "Therapeutic Potential and Mechanisms of Berberine in Cardiovascular Disease." Current Pharmacology Reports 2.6 (2016): 281–292. and

26) Jeong, Hyun Woo, et al. "Berberine suppresses proinflammatory responses through AMPK activation in macrophages." American Journal of Physiology-Endocrinology and Metabolism 296.4 (2009)

27) Lau, Chi-Wai, et al. "Cardiovascular actions of berberine." Cardiovascular Drug Reviews 19.3 (2001): 234–244.

28) Zhang, Ming, et al. "Therapeutic Potential and Mechanisms of Berberine in Cardiovascular Disease." Current Pharmacology Reports 2.6 (2016): 281–292.

29) Nutrition Review Drug-free Alternatives for Arrhythmia April 19, 2013 By Jim English

30) Coccimiglio, John, et al. "Antioxidant, Antibacterial, and Cytotoxic Activities of the Ethanolic Origanum vulgare Extract and Its Major Constituents." (2016).

31) Dinda, Biswanath, et al. "Therapeutic potentials of baicalin and its aglycone, baicalein against inflammatory disorders." European journal of medicinal chemistry 131 (2017): 68–80.

32) Gao, Li, et al. "A bioinformatic approach for the discovery of antiaging effects of baicalein from Scutellaria baicalensis Georgi." *Rejuvenation research* 19.5 (2016): 414–422.

33) Chan, Shih-Hung, et al. "Baicalein is an available anti-atherosclerotic compound through modulation of nitric oxide-related mechanism under oxLDL exposure." *Oncotarget* 7.28 (2016): 42881.

34) Kim, Ohn Soon, et al. "Extracts of Scutellariae Radix inhibit low-density lipoprotein oxidation and the lipopolysaccharide-induced macrophage inflammatory response." *Molecular medicine reports* 12.1 (2015): 1335–1341.

35) Kim, Ohn Soon, et al. "Extracts of Scutellariae Radix inhibit low-density lipoprotein oxidation and the lipopolysaccharide-induced macrophage inflammatory response." *Molecular medicine reports* 12.1 (2015): 1335–1341.

36) Liu, Hui, et al. "The Fascinating Effects of Baicalein on Cancer: A Review." International Journal of Molecular Sciences 17.10 (2016): 1681.

37) Wu, Xue, et al. "Advances of wogonin, an extract from Scutellaria baicalensis, for the treatment of multiple tumors." OncoTargets and therapy 9 (2016): 2935.

38) Lee, Donghyun, et al. "Use of Baicalin-Conjugated Gold Nanoparticles for Apoptotic Induction of Breast Cancer Cells." *Nanoscale Research Letters* 11.1 (2016): 381.

39) Wei, L., et al. "Oroxylin A induces dissociation of hexokinase II from the mitochondria and inhibits glycolysis by SIRT3-mediated deacetylation of cyclophilin D in breast carcinoma." Cell death & disease 4.4 (2013): e601.

40) Wei, L., et al. "Oroxylin A inhibits glycolysis-dependent proliferation of human breast cancer via promoting SIRT3-mediated SOD2 transcription and HIF1α destabilization." *Cell death & disease* 6.4 (2015): e1714.

41) Wang, Ke, et al. "Curcumin inhibits aerobic glycolysis and induces mitochondrial-mediated apoptosis through hexokinase II in human colorectal cancer cells in vitro." Anti-cancer drugs 26.1 (2015): 15–24.

42) Sun, Yu, et al. "Oroxylin A suppresses invasion through down-regulating the expression of matrix metalloproteinase-2/9 in MDA-MB-435 human breast cancer cells." European journal of pharmacology 603.1–3 (2009): 22–28.

43) Li, Hua-Nan, et al. "Apoptosis induction of oroxylin A in human cervical cancer HeLa cell line in vitro and in vivo." Toxicology 257.1 (2009): 80–85.

44) Yang, Yong, et al. "Oroxylin A induces G2/M phase cell-cycle arrest via inhibiting Cdk7-mediated expression of Cdc2/p34 in human gastric carcinoma BGC-823 cells." Journal of Pharmacy and Pharmacology 60.11 (2008): 1459–1463.

45) Hu, Yang, et al. "Oroxylin A induced apoptosis of human hepatocellular carcinoma cell line HepG2 was involved in its antitumor activity." Biochemical and biophysical research communications 351.2 (2006): 521–527.

46) Gao, Ying, et al. "Oroxylin A inhibits angiogenesis through blocking vascular endothelial growth factor-induced KDR/Flk-1 phosphorylation." Journal of cancer research and clinical oncology 136.5 (2010): 667–675.

47) Mu, Rong, et al. "Involvement of p53 in oroxylin A-induced apoptosis in cancer cells." Molecular carcinogenesis 48.12 (2009): 1159–1169.

48) Yao, Jing, et al. "Oroxylin a prevents inflammation-related tumor through down-regulation of inflammatory gene expression by inhibiting NF-κB signaling." Molecular carcinogenesis 53.2 (2014): 145–158.

49) Hsieh, Y., et al. "The lipoxygenase inhibitor, baicalein, modulates cell adhesion and migration by up-regulation of integrins and vinculin in rat heart endothelial cells." British journal of pharmacology 151.8 (2007): 1235–1245.

50) Song, Xiuming, et al. "Oroxylin A, a classical natural product, shows a novel inhibitory effect on angiogenesis induced by lipopolysaccharide." Pharmacological Reports 64.5 (2012): 1189–1199.

51) Tseng, Tzu-Ling, et al. "Oroxylin-A rescues LPS-induced acute lung injury via regulation of NF-κB signaling pathway in rodents." PLoS One 7.10 (2012): e47403.

52) Wang, Hong, et al. "An estrogen receptor dependent mechanism of Oroxylin A in the repression of inflammatory response." PloS one 8.7 (2013): e69555.

53) Ye, Fei, et al. "Molecular mechanism of anti-prostate cancer activity of Scutellaria baicalensis extract." Nutrition and cancer 57.1 (2007): 100–110.

54) Moore, Jessy, Michael Yousef, and Evangelia Tsiani. "Anticancer effects of rosemary (Rosmarinus officinalis L.) extract and rosemary extract polyphenols." Nutrients 8.11 (2016): 731.

55) Olszanecki, R., et al. "Effect of curcumin on atherosclerosis in apoE/LDLR-double knockout mice." Journal of physiology and pharmacology: an official journal of the Polish Physiological Society 56.4 (2005): 627–635.

Coronary Calcium Score
Benefits of Aged Garlic

JIM HAS AN ELEVATED CORONARY calcium score in the 95th percentile, indicating a high risk for future heart attack. He is being treated by his cardiologist with daily aspirin and atorvastatin, a statin drug to reduce cholesterol.

Currently, we are following a number of similar patients with elevated coronary calcium score who are being treated with statin drugs by their cardiologist. The elevated calcium score indicates a higher risk for a future coronary event, such as chest pain, angina, heart attack, etc. Current cardiology dogma dictates that these patients should be treated with statin drugs to lower their cholesterol, thus preventing heart disease.

Cholesterol Theory Shown to Be False

The problem with this cardiology dogma is that the cholesterol theory of atherosclerotic disease has been shown to be false by many studies. These studies have been nicely summarized by Dr. Ware of the University of Ontario. (9) Dr. Ware's fine article in *Medical Hypotheses* (2009), reveals that both autopsy and coronary-calcium-score studies fail to show a correlation between serum cholesterol and the amount of atherosclerotic plaque. Thus, the theory that elevated cholesterol causes hardening of the arteries is essentially proven false.

Statin Drugs Disappointing for Calcium Score

Two randomized trials using statin drugs to reduce calcium scores showed disappointing results. (10,11) In Dr. E. S. Houslay's trial, published in 2006 in *Heart*, 102 patients were randomized and treated for two years with either 80 mg/d of atorvastatin (a statin drug) or a placebo. (10) As expected, the statin-treated group had a 53% reduction in LDL cholesterol, while the placebo group had no change in theirs. Although the researchers were expecting a calcium-score benefit from the statin treatment, they found the opposite. Paradoxically, the statin group had *greater increase* in calcium score (26%) than the placebo group (only 18%). The authors concluded that

> *statin treatment does not have a major effect on the rate of progression of coronary artery calcification. (10)*

The second trial, by Dr. Axel Schmermund, reported in *Circulation* (2006), randomized 471 patients with no pre-existing coronary artery disease and treated them for one year with either low-dose (10mg/d) or high-dose (80 mg/d) atorvastatin therapy. In the high-dose group (80 mg/d), the LDL cholesterol was reduced from 106 to 87 mg/dL, an approximately 20% reduction. However, the low-dose statin group had no change in LDL cholesterol from baseline (108 vs 109 mg/dL). The authors were expecting a reduction in the progression of calcium scores in the high-dose statin group, with a 20% reduction in LDL cholesterol. They were surprised to find no difference in calcium scores between the two groups. The high-dose atorvastatin group actually had slightly greater progression of calcium score (27%) vs. (25%) for the low-dose group. The authors concluded:

> *Coronary artery calcification (CAC) progression showed no relationship with on-treatment LDL cholesterol levels. (11)*

According to Dr. Edward A. Gill, Professor of Cardiology at University of Colorado, writing in 2010 in *Current Atherosclerosis Reports,* statins are no better than a placebo:

All five prospective studies and now most recent observational trials find that HMG-CoA reductase therapy [i.e., statin drug therapy] does not result in regression of coronary calcium; in fact, the rate of progression is not different than placebo treatment. (45)

What Interventions Have Been Successful to Reduce Calcium Score?

As we can see from the above studies, statin drugs are quite effective for lowering cholesterol, yet fail to reduce or slow progression of the calcium score. The sad truth is that mainstream cardiology offers no effective treatment for slowing progression of the calcium score. Perhaps we should look elsewhere for such a treatment modality. Dr. Budoff explored the use of aged garlic in slowing progression of calcium score in three studies. (1–3)

Aged Garlic for Calcium Score

In Dr. Budoff 's first study, published in 2006 in the *Journal of Nutrition*, 23 "high-risk" patients maintained on a stable dose of statin drug and aspirin were divided at random and given either a placebo or 4 mL of aged garlic (1200 mg Kyolic Aged Garlic Liquid). After one year of treatment, the aged garlic group showed a 7.5% progression in their calcium score, considerably lower than the 22.2% progression in the placebo group. (1) Remember that both groups were maintained on statin drugs during the one-year follow-up, and cholesterol levels were the same for both groups.

In a second study by Dr. Budoff, published in *Preventive Medicine* in 2009, sixty-five "intermediate risk" patients, all maintained on statins, were randomized and treated for one year with either a placebo or aged garlic extract (250 mg). (2) In addition, the garlic group was given the following vitamins (the product used was Kyolic 108 Aged Garlic by Wakunaga) (2):

- Vitamin B12 (100 microg)
- Folic acid (300 microg)
- Vitamin B6 (12.5 mg)
- L-arginine (100 mg)

After one year of treatment, the aged garlic group had significantly less coronary artery calcification progression (6.8%) compared to the placebo group (26.5%).

A third study by Dr. Budoff in 2012 in the *Journal of Cardiovascular Research* randomized 65 firefighters and treated one group with aged garlic plus Co-Q-10 (Kyolic Aged Garlic-Co-Q10 Formula 110, Wakunaga) and the other a placebo. (3) About 25% of the Aged Garlic+CoQ10 were on statins and 31% of placebo group were on statins. After one year of treatment, the aged garlic group showed less progression of calcium score (32 vs. 58 absolute) and (18.9% vs 27.4%). C-reactive protein (CRP) was also lower in the garlic group.

A 2015 report by Dr. Budoff in the *Journal of Nutrition and Food Sciences* pooled four placebo-controlled, double-blind, randomized studies with 210 patients, (182 of whom completed the study). All had calcium score, at baseline and at 12 months. At 1 year, median calcium score progression was significantly lower in the AGE (aged garlic extract) group, (10.8) than the placebo group (18.3). There were no differences in serum cholesterol or CRP levels between the groups. (30)

Additional Benefits of Garlic

In a 2013 study by Dr. Kumar, garlic was found beneficial as an adjunct to Metformin 500 mg twice a day in obese diabetics. (12) Garlic lowers blood pressure and has been found useful in hypertensive patients. (13) In addition, garlic is useful as an anti-microbial agent (4–8).

Garlic Reduces Calcium Score Progression: Mechanism of Action

Other chapters in this book discuss the limitations of the cholesterol hypothesis, recent revelations about atherosclerotic plaque as infected biofilm, and its association with increased gut permeability, also called "leaky gut." This would certainly explain our somewhat paradoxical findings in the three studies by Dr. Budoff showing that garlic is more effective than statin drugs. A natural antimicrobial agent, the lowly garlic bulb shows the ability to retard progression of calcium score, in contrast to statin drugs, dogmatically offered by mainstream cardiology. Even though they reduce cholesterol, statins have no benefit for calcium score.

Garlic as Anti-Microbial Agent

Although various mechanisms have been proposed to explain the benefits of garlic in cardiovascular disease, I would like to focus on garlic as an anti-microbial agent. (4–8) Unlike conventional antibiotics, which may disrupt the normal intestinal flora, garlic's antimicrobial properties act against pathogenic gut bacteria with relative sparing of the beneficial "friendly" gut bacteria. (4) Or, in other words, as Dr. Leyla Bayan (2014) says, *"Garlic exerts a differential inhibition between beneficial intestinal microflora and potentially harmful enterobacteria."* (4)

Dr. Rees studied Garlic's antimicrobial activity, finding broad-spectrum activity against *"many bacteria, yeasts, fungi and virus. All micro-organisms tested were susceptible to Garlic."* (5) Dr. Angela Filocamo in 2012 studied garlic in a bacterial population that is representative of the colonic microbiota. Lactobacillus was more resistant to garlic than clostridium, a gram-positive bacteria that includes pathogenic forms. The author suggested the *"consumption [of garlic] may favor the growth of these beneficial bacterial species in the gut. Garlic intake has the potential to temporarily modulate the gut microbiota."* (6) A full discussion of the antimicrobial spectrum of garlic can be found in an excellent article in 2015 by Dr. Packia Lekshmi. (7) Mark Slevin's 2012 article reported on natural products with vascular protective properties and significant anti-atherogenic potential. Dr. Slevin mentions aged garlic, resveratrol, and green tea extract (ECGC) as the most promising. (8)

Pseudomonas Biofilm in Atherosclerotic Plaque Material

Dr. Bernard Lanter studied atherosclerotic plaque and was able to identify Pseudomonas 16S rRNA genes in 6 of 15 cases. (14) The virulence of Pseudomonas is attributed to "quorum sensing," the ability of these bacterial cells to communicate with one another to form biofilms. (16) Dr. Thomas Bjarnsholt considers disruption of this quorum sensing to be the key to controlling pseudomonas biofilm infections. That is exactly what garlic does. In vitro and in vivo animal studies show that garlic inhibits quorum sensing and therefore the virulence of pseudomonas. (15) An excellent way to study the effect of allicin, the active ingredient in garlic, on the pseudomonas organism is to tag the bacteria with the green fluorescent protein (GFP), a protein that was first isolated in the jellyfish. The results of an elegant series of in vitro experiments using allicin-treated and GFP-modified Pseudomonas organisms published in 2013 by Dr. Lin Lihua's group (17) showed the following:

Allicin treatment not only reduced the adhesion ratio of P. aeruginosa, but also inhibited EPS (extracellular polysaccharide) secretion and down-regulates production of some Quorum Sensing -controlled virulence factors. These results imply that allicin can disturb the formation and maturation of P. aeruginosa biofilm, and suggest that allicin may represent a promising therapeutic candidate for the management of P. aeruginosa biofilms. (17)

Polymicrobial Colonization

Others have found diverse colonies of bacterial, fungal, and protozoal life-forms colonizing biofilms in arterial plaque. (18–20) In view of this, it would be useful to investigate other botanical agents with known antimicrobial activity, such as olive-leaf extract, oregano oil, and berberine. Perhaps a combination of such natural products would have a more powerful synergistic effect than any of them acting alone. This would be a fertile area for future research.

Other Agents to Disrupt Biofilm: EDTA, Proteolytic Enzymes, and Reactive Oxygen

Other agents that disrupt biofilm to consider for future study include EDTA, proteolytic enzymes, and reactive oxygen. Dr. Zhenqiu Liu found that EDTA enhanced the effect of antibiotics against pseudomonas biofilm, therefore suggesting it might be effective in reversing or slowing progression of the calcium score and the atherosclerotic process. We await these further studies. (31)

Proteolytic enzymes (enzymes that break down proteins and peptides) have been found useful for disrupting biofilm-forming infections in various locations in the body. (33–38) Reactive oxygen in various forms, hyperbaric oxygen, ozone, etc., have been found useful for treating biofilm-forming infections. (39–44)

Garlic Reduces Plaque in Genetically Modified Mice

The benefits of garlic on slowing calcium-score progression are well established. What about garlic for preventing plaque formation itself? This question was studied in atherosclerotic mice by Ayelet Gonen's group at the Institute of Lipid and Atherosclerosis Research, Sheba Medical Center, Tel Hashomer Israel. (21) Dr. Gonen studied the effect of daily treatment with allicin (the active ingredient in garlic) on mice that had been genetically modified to form atherosclerotic plaque in the aortic sinus. These were ApoE-knockout mice, and LDL receptor knockout mice. Daily allicin (9 mg/kg) reduced the atherosclerotic plaque area by 70% in apoE-deficient mice, and by 60% in LDL receptor knockout mice. (21) This is rather impressive. They went further, showing that allicin binds directly to the LDL particle, preventing LDL oxidation, and inhibits macrophage uptake and degradation of the LDL particles. The authors speculated this is the mechanism for atherosclerosis prevention using garlic.

Future Research Experiments

As mentioned above, independent researchers have found polymicrobial organisms colonizing biofilms in atherosclerotic plaque. One question I have is this: *Why not conduct a series of experiments using these same techniques to look for infected biofilms in the atherosclerotic plaque material in animal models of atherosclerosis ?* Perhaps the Institute of Lipid and Atherosclerosis Research might collaborate and share mouse plaque specimens with Drs. Stephen Fry, Bernard Lanter, and Stephan Ott. This would answer a number of important questions. What is the timing of the infection in the plaque? Is infection a prerequisite for plaque formation. Is the infection a later event? Does infection seed the plaque after plaque formation? Exactly when in the life cycle of the atherosclerotic plaque does the infection occur? Is garlic's preventive mechanism solely a result of preventing LDL oxidation and inhibiting macrophage uptake, as Dr. Gonen speculates ? Or does infection also play a role in these supposedly "pristine" animal models of knockout mice genetically bred to form atherosclerosis ? These and other questions could be answered by studying plaque from animal models using the 16s RNA cloning and fluorescent-imaging techniques used in the labs of Drs. Lanter, Ott and Fry.

Eliminate Wheat: Benefits of a Gluten-Free Diet

Dr. William Davis, cardiologist from Wisconsin, brought attention to the adverse effects of wheat consumption in his book, *Wheat Belly,* a *New York Times* bestseller, and his later book, *Undoctored.* Dr. Davis strongly recommends a wheat-free diet for those patients with elevated calcium score as part of diet and lifestyle modification, a cornerstone of the calcium-score reduction program. (24–26)

Our Program for Elevated Calcium Score:

- Aged garlic
- MK-4 and MK-7 versions of vitamin K2

- Berberine
- Co-Q10
- L-arginine
- Resveratrol, pterostilbene
- Homocysteine-reducing program (B6, B12, methylfolate)
- Linus Pauling Protocol (lysine, proline, vitamin C, tocotrienols, MK-7 vit K2)
- William Davis Track Your Plaque Protocol (niacin, omega-3 fish oil, vitamin D3, vitamin K2, eliminate wheat products)
- Weight reduction
- Hormone optimization (optimize thyroid, testosterone, estrogen progesterone)
- Heal the leaky gut (probiotics, glutamine, colostrum)
- Eliminate NSAIDS and PPIs, which cause dysbiosis and leaky gut.
- Eliminate pesticides, glyphosate and GMO food, eat organic.

♦　♦　♦　♦　♦

◆ References for Chapter 8

1) Budoff, Matthew. "Aged garlic extract retards progression of coronary artery calcification." *The Journal of Nutrition* 136.3 (2006): 741S-744S.

2) Budoff, M. J., et al. "Aged garlic extract supplemented with B vitamins, folic acid and L-arginine retards the progression of subclinical atherosclerosis: a randomized clinical trial." *Preventive medicine* 49.2–3 (2009): 101.

3) Zeb, Irfan, Budoff M et al. "Aged Garlic Extract and Coenzyme Q10 Have Favorable Effect on Inflammatory Markers and Coronary Atherosclerosis Progression: A Randomized Clinical Trial." *Journal of Cardiovascular Disease Research* 3.3 (2012): 185–190. PMC. Web. 11 June 2015.

4) Bayan, Leyla, Peir Hossain Koulivand, and Ali Gorji. "Garlic: A Review of Potential Therapeutic Effects." *Avicenna Journal of Phytomedicine* 4.1 (2014): 1–14. Print.

5) Rees, L. P., et al. "A quantitative assessment of the antimicrobial activity of garlic (Allium sativum)." *World Journal of Microbiology and Biotechnology* 9.3 (1993): 303–307.

6) Filocamo, Angela, et al. "Effect of garlic powder on the growth of commensal bacteria from the gastrointestinal tract." *Phytomedicine* 19.8 (2012): 707–711.

7) Packia Lekshmi, N. C. J., et al. "Antimicrobial Spectrum of Allium Species–A Review." *History* 15.44 (2015): 1–5.

8) Slevin, Mark, et al. "Unique vascular protective properties of natural products: supplements or future main-line drugs with significant anti-atherosclerotic potential." *Vasc Cell* 4.1 (2012): 9.

9) Ware, William R. "The mainstream hypothesis that LDL cholesterol drives atherosclerosis may have been falsified by non-invasive imaging of coronary artery plaque burden and progression." *Medical hypotheses* 73.4 (2009): 596–600.

10) Houslay, E S et al. "Progressive Coronary Calcification despite Intensive Lipid-lowering Treatment: A Randomised Controlled Trial." *Heart* 92.9 (2006): 1207–1212. PMC. Web. 11 June 2015.

11) Schmermund, Axel, et al. "Effect of Intensive Versus Standard Lipid-Lowering Treatment With Atorvastatin on the Progression of Calcified Coronary Atherosclerosis Over 12 Months A Multicenter, Randomized, Double-Blind Trial." *Circulation* 113.3 (2006): 427–437.

12) Kumar, Rahat et al. "Antihyperglycemic, Antihyperlipidemic, Anti-Inflammatory and Adenosine Deaminase– Lowering Effects of Garlic in Patients with Type 2 Diabetes Mellitus with Obesity." *Diabetes, Metabolic Syndrome and Obesity: Targets and Therapy* 6 (2013): 49–56. PMC. Web. 12 June 2015.

13) Xiong, X. J., et al. "Garlic for hypertension: A systematic review and meta-analysis of randomized controlled trials." *Phytomedicine* 22.3 (2015): 352–361.

14) Lanter, Bernard B., Karin Sauer, and David G. Davies. "Bacteria present in carotid arterial plaques are found as biofilm deposits which may contribute to enhanced risk of plaque rupture." *MBio* 5.3 (2014): e01206–14.

15) Harjai, K., R. Kumar, and S. Singh. "Garlic blocks quorum sensing and attenuates the virulence of Pseudomonas aeruginosa." *FEMS immunology and medical microbiology* 58.2 (2010): 161.

16) Bjarnsholt, Thomas, and Michael Givskov. "The role of quorum sensing in the pathogenicity of the cunning aggressor Pseudomonas aeruginosa." *Analytical and bioanalytical chemistry* 387.2 (2007): 409–414.

17) Lihua, Lin, et al. "Effects of allicin on the formation of Pseudomonas aeruginosabiofinm and the production of quorum-sensing controlled virulence factors." *Pol J Microbiol* 62 (2013): 243–51.

18) Ott, Stephan J., et al. "Detection of diverse bacterial signatures in atherosclerotic lesions of patients with coronary heart disease." *Circulation* 113.7 (2006): 929–937.

19) Ott, S. J., et al. "Fungal rDNA signatures in coronary atherosclerotic_Ott_2007_ Athrosclerosis Fungal rDNA signatures in coronary atherosclerotic plaques." *Environmental microbiology* 9.12 (2007): 3035–3045.

20) Fry, Stephen Eugene, et al. "Putative biofilm-forming organisms in the human vasculature: expanded case reports and review of the literature." *Phlebological Review* 22.1 (2014): 24–37.

21) Gonen, Ayelet, et al. "The antiatherogenic effect of allicin: possible mode of action." *Pathobiology* 72.6 (2005): 325–334.

22) Gonen, Ayelet, et al. "The antiatherogenic effect of allicin: possible mode of action." *Pathobiology* 72.6 (2005): 325–334

24) Statin scare By Dr. Davis | May 23, 2016

25) The Wheat Belly lifestyle BEGAN with heart health. By Dr. Davis | September 15, 2015

26) My Wheat Belly turning point By Dr. Davis | June 11, 2015

27) Hom, Christopher, Matthew Budoff, and Yanting Luo. "The effects of aged garlic extract on coronary artery calcification progression and blood pressure." *Journal of the American College of Cardiology* 65.10 Supplement (2015): A1472.

28) Rao, P. S. S., et al. "Diallyl sulfide: potential use in novel therapeutic interventions in alcohol, drugs, and disease mediated cellular toxicity by targeting cytochrome P450 2E1." Current drug metabolism 16.6 (2015): 486.

29) Matsumoto, Suguru, et al. "Aged Garlic Extract Reduces Low Attenuation Plaque in Coronary Arteries of Patients with Metabolic Syndrome in a Prospective Randomized Double-Blind Study–3." *The Journal of nutrition* 146.2 (2016): 427S-432S.

30) Hom C, Luo Y, Budoff MJ (2015) The Effects of Aged Garlic Extract on Coronary Artery Calcification Progression. *J Nutr Food Sci* S5:005.

31) Liu, Zhenqiu, et al. "In vitro and in vivo activity of EDTA and antibacterial agents against the biofilm of mucoid Pseudomonas aeruginosa." *Infection* 45.1 (2017): 23–31.

32) Mukherji, R., A. Patil, and A. Prabhune. "Role of extracellular proteases in biofilm disruption of gram positive bacteria with special emphasis on Staphylococcus aureus biofilms." *Enz Eng* 4 (2015): 126.

33) Banar, Maryam, et al. "Evaluation of mannosidase and trypsin enzymes effects on biofilm production of Pseudomonas aeruginosa isolated from burn wound infections." *PloS one* 11.10 (2016): e0164622.

34) Molobela, I. Phyllis, T. Eugene Cloete, and Mervyn Beukes. "Protease and amylase enzymes for biofilm removal and degradation of extracellular polymeric substances (EPS) produced by Pseudomonas fluorescens bacteria." *African Journal of Microbiology Research* 4.14 (2010): 1515–1524.

35) Drilling, Amanda J., et al. "Fighting sinus-derived Staphylococcus aureus biofilms in vitro with a bacteriophage-derived muralytic enzyme." *International forum of allergy & rhinology*. Vol. 6. No. 4. 2016.

36) Al-Khateeb, T. H., and Y. Nusair. "Effect of the proteolytic enzyme serrapeptase on swelling, pain and trismus after surgical extraction of mandibular third molars." *International journal of oral and maxillofacial surgery* 37.3 (2008): 264–268.

37) Shahid S. Role of Systemic Enzymes in Infections. WebmedCentral COMPLEMENTARY MEDICINE 2012;3(1):WMC002504

38) Tiwari, Manju. "The role of serratiopeptidase in the resolution of inflammation." Asian journal of pharmaceutical sciences 12.3 (2017): 209–215.

39) Dryden, M. S., et al. "Reactive oxygen: a novel antimicrobial mechanism for targeting biofilm-associated infection." Journal of global antimicrobial resistance (2017).

40) Memar, Mohammad Yousef, et al. "Antimicrobial use of reactive oxygen therapy: current insights." Infection and drug resistance 11 (2018): 567.

41) Bialoszewski, Dariusz, et al. "Activity of ozonated water and ozone against Staphylococcus aureus and Pseudomonas aeruginosa biofilms." Medical science monitor: international medical journal of experimental and clinical research 17.11 (2011): BR339.

42) Koyama, Ryouta, et al. "Antimicrobial and Antibiofilm Effects of Ozonated Water for Prevention and Treatment of Bone and Joint Infections." Journal of St. Marianna University 6.1 (2015): 1–7.

43) Song, Mingsheng, et al. "The antibacterial effect of topical ozone on the treatment of MRSA skin infection." Molecular medicine reports 17.2 (2018): 2449–2455.

44) Delgado-Roche, Livan, Gregorio Martínez-Sánchez, and Lamberto Re. "Ozone oxidative preconditioning prevents atherosclerosis development in New Zealand white rabbits." Journal of cardiovascular pharmacology 61.2 (2013): 160–165.

45) Gill, Edward A. "Does statin therapy affect the progression of atherosclerosis measured by a coronary calcium score?." *Current atherosclerosis reports* 12.2 (2010): 83–87.

Vitamin K: Is There Anything It Can't Do ?

IN 1973, IN MY SECOND-YEAR of medical school, we made rounds every morning on the medical ward at the University of Illinois Hospital. A five-milligram injection of **Vitamin K** was commonly ordered for liver disease patients with bleeding disorders. Later, when I did my three-month rotation on the surgical floor, I found surgeons pacing impatiently whenever their procedures where delayed. The delay was usually due to an abnormal coagulation profile from a blood-thinner medication called warfarin, which antagonizes vitamin K and inhibits clotting. A vitamin K injection promptly restores the coagulation factors, and the procedure can proceed. Thankfully, the surgeons then stop pacing back and forth, and happily head to the operating room.

More Than Just Clotting Factors

New research into cell physiology over the last two decades shows that the K (koagulation) vitamin has other, more extensive benefits. Vitamin K is involved in the activation of vitamin K-dependent (VKD) proteins. Activation involves "carboxylation" (adding carbon dioxide), which renders VKD proteins active in roles that include "hemostasis, apoptosis, bone mineralization, calcium homeostasis, growth control, and signal transduction." Further studies show that although we may have sufficient vitamin K intake to prevent bleeding disorders, because of the "triage effect" described by Vermeer, we don't take in enough Vitamin K to prevent the degenerative diseases of aging, atherosclerosis with arterial calcification, osteoporosis, and cancer.

(5,6)(25)(37) Dr. Cees Vermeer of the Netherlands says in 2011 *Menopause International*:

> *It seems, however, that our dietary vitamin K intake is too low to support the carboxylation of at least some of these Gla-proteins. According to the triage theory, long-term vitamin K inadequacy is an independent, but modifiable risk factor for the development of degenerative diseases of ageing, including osteoporosis and atherosclerosis. (6)*

Soft-Tissue and Coronary Artery Calcification

It is well known based on clinical experience alone that warfarin, a vitamin K antagonist, increases soft-tissue and arterial calcifications. Human studies confirm increased vascular calcification is induced by warfarin. In addition, this warfarin effect is reversible with high Vitamin K intake. One might then expect increased coronary artery calcification in patients with low vitamin K intake. Indeed, an association between low vitamin K intake and increased risk for coronary artery disease was found in the Rotterdam Study (1–5).

Discordant Warfarin Calcium Scoring Studies

Calcium scoring studies in patients on warfarin fail to confirm increased coronary artery calcification from warfarin use. I suspect there is some error in these studies. Perhaps the control patients had vitamin K deficiency and formed coronary artery calcification at levels similar to those of the warfarin-treated group, thus explaining the negative studies.

Good Correlation with Matrix GLA

As one might expect, serial calcium score studies by Dr. Kyla Shea showed benefit for calcium score in vitamin-K-treated patients. (43) Thus, we can recommend vitamin K as part of a program to reduce calcium score annual progression and reduce risk for myocardial infarction (heart attack).

A number of excellent studies done by Drs. Vermeer et al. from the Netherlands showed an excellent correlation between calcium score, heart-disease risk, mortality from heart disease, and uncarboxylated Matrix GLA protein, the best marker for Vitamin K deficiency. (5,6)(25)(37)

An excellent calcium scoring study by Drs. Vermeer and Roger Rennenberg showed good correlation between calcium score and vitamin K status. (11) Remember, vitamin K is an essential cofactor to carboxylate matrix Gla protein, itself a potent inhibitor of vascular calcification. Dr. Vermeer found that calcium score was significantly associated with ucMGP (uncarboxylated Matrix GLA, an indicator of Vitamin K deficiency). (11)

Another study by Dr. Ellen Van den Heuvel published in *Maturitas* in 2013, again showed a more than two-fold increase in cardiovascular risk for elderly men and women with lower vitamin K status, as measured by the amount of uncarboxylated MGP. (44)

Another Vermeer study published in *Atherosclerosis* in July 2014, showed a more than doubling of mortality in the low vitamin K group. This study followed 800 people for 5 years with a mean age of 65, all with known cardiovascular disease. Patients in the highest quartile for uncarboxylated Matrix GLA (uMGLA), a marker for low vitamin K status, had almost double the mortality from cardiovascular disease. (45) More recent studies show vitamin K2 slows or prevents coronary artery calcification in animal models and renal dialysis patients (39–41)

Calcium supplementation, as you might expect, increases the risk of myocardial infarction. (5) This is best explained by underlying vitamin K deficiency in patients taking vitamin D and calcium for osteoporosis prevention. Obviously, adding in Vitamin K is useful here.

Preventing and Treating Cancer

Another surprising benefit of Vitamin K is that is can serve as a potent anti-cancer treatment. (32–36) A number of cell culture and animal xenograft studies show that vitamin K2 induces "apoptosis" (programmed cell death) in cancer cells. (12–21) A number of different cancers were studied, including glioblastoma, hepatocellular cancer, lung cancer, and prostate cancer. (12–21)

Based on these reports, one might include vitamin K2 (45 mg per day) to a program for prevention of cancer recurrence after treatment. (28–31) Vitamin K2 has been studied and found effective for inducing apoptosis in ovarian cancer, leukemia, and breast-cancer cell lines. MK-4 and MK7 are the two versions of K2. MK-7 has the longer side chain, called "Geranylgeraniol," which has potent anti-cancer activity. (38)

Vitamin K2 for Myelodysplastic Syndrome

A dreaded adverse toxic effect of repeated chemotherapy treatments is bone marrow failure. This is called myelodysplastic syndrome, in which the patient's bone marrow is unable to make platelets and blood cells. At this stage, further chemotherapy is deemed futile, and without weekly platelet and red cell transfusions, the patient would not survive. Dr. Takami reported in 1999 successful therapy of myelodysplastic syndrome with Vitamin K2, 45 mg a day.(47)

Vitamin K for Rheumatoid Arthritis

Another study shows Vitamin K is useful as a treatment for Rheumatoid arthritis. (22)

Vitamin K for Bone Mineral Density

For women taking Calcium and Vitamin D to maintain strong bones and prevent osteoporosis, vitamin K is especially important. In the past few years, many bone-calcium supplement companies have added Vitamin K to upgrade their calcium and vitamin D product. Vitamin K strengthens bones, increases bone mineral density (BMD), and reduces fracture risk. Retrospective studies of Vitamin K antagonists, coumarin type blood thinners suggest an adverse effect on vertebral BMD and fracture risk. (24)

In a randomized trial using dual energy X-ray absorptiometry, known as DEXA, Vermeer showed that K2 improved bone mineral content (BMC) and femoral neck width, (but not bone mineral density). (25)

Vitamin K for Nausea and Vomiting of Pregnancy

A 1952 report by Dr. Merkel appeared in a mainstream obstetrics journal on the use of combined vitamin K and vitamin C for relief of nausea and vomiting of pregnancy. (46) Thanks and credit to Jonathan Wright's Newsletter for bringing this to my attention (June 2015).

Which Version of Vitamin K is Best?

Some authors suggest the long-chain natto derived MK7 version is more potent and preferable to MK4 version of vitamin K2. (37) So, it might be prudent to take a K2 formulation that includes both MK4 and MK7 versions. Dr. Elke Theuwissen says in a 2012 article:

Later studies, in which the long-chain menaquinone-7 (MK-7) was used to counteract warfarin-induced calcification, showed that this form of menaquinone was even more potent than menaquinone-4. This is consistent with population-based studies in which only the long-chain menaquinones had cardioprotective effects." (37)

♦ ♦ ♦ ♦ ♦

♦ References for Chapter 9

1) Seyama, Y., et al. "Effect of vitamin K2 on experimental calcinosis induced by vitamin D2 in rat soft tissue." International journal for vitamin and nutrition research. Internationale Zeitschrift fur Vitamin-und Ernahrungsforschung. Journal international de vitaminologie et de nutrition 66.1 (1996): 36–38.

2) Kawashima, Hidetoshi, et al. "Effects of vitamin K2 (menatetrenone) on atherosclerosis and blood coagulation in hypercholesterolemic rabbits." The Japanese Journal of Pharmacology 75.2 (1997): 135–143.

3) Beulens, Joline WJ, et al. "High dietary menaquinone intake is associated with reduced coronary calcification." Atherosclerosis 203.2 (2009): 489–493.

4) Gast, Gerrie-Cor M., et al. "A high menaquinone intake reduces the incidence of coronary heart disease." Nutrition, Metabolism and Cardiovascular Diseases 19.7 (2009): 504–510.

5) Vermeer, Cees Vermeer. "Vitamin K: the effect on health beyond coagulation–an overview." Food & nutrition research 56.1 (2012): 5329.

6) Vermeer, Cees, and Elke Theuwissen. "Vitamin K, osteoporosis and degenerative diseases of ageing." Menopause international 17.1 (2011): 19–23.

7) McCann, Joyce C., and Bruce N. Ames. "Vitamin K, an example of triage theory: is micronutrient inadequacy linked to diseases of aging?–." The American journal of clinical nutrition 90.4 (2009): 889–907.

8 Berkner, K. L., and K. W. Runge. "The physiology of vitamin K nutriture and vitamin K-dependent protein function in atherosclerosis." Journal of Thrombosis and Haemostasis 2.12 (2004): 2118–2132.

9) Seyama, Y., et al. "Effect of vitamin K2 on experimental calcinosis induced by vitamin D2 in rat soft tissue." International journal for vitamin and nutrition research. Internationale Zeitschrift fur Vitamin-und Ernahrungsforschung. Journal international de vitaminologie et de nutrition 66.1 (1996): 36–38.

10) Kawashima, Hidetoshi, et al. "Effects of vitamin K2 (menatetrenone) on atherosclerosis and blood coagulation in hypercholesterolemic rabbits." The Japanese Journal of Pharmacology 75.2 (1997): 135–143.

11) Rennenberg, Roger JMW, et al. "Calcium scores and matrix Gla protein levels: association with vitamin K status." European journal of clinical investigation 40.4 (2010): 344–349.

12) Mizuta, Toshihiko, et al. "The effect of menatetrenone, a vitamin K2 analog, on disease recurrence and survival in patients with hepatocellular carcinoma after curative treatment." *Cancer* 106.4 (2006): 867–872.

13) Zhong, Jian-Hong, et al. "Postoperative use of the chemopreventive vitamin K2 analog in patients with hepatocellular carcinoma." *PloS one* 8.3 (2013): e58082.

14) Kuriyama, Shigeki, et al. "Vitamins K2, K3 and K5 exert in vivo antitumor effects on hepatocellular carcinoma by regulating the expression of G1 phase-related cell cycle molecules." *International journal of oncology* 27.2 (2005): 505–511.

15) Oztopcu, Pinar, et al. "Comparison of vitamins K~ 1, K~ 2 and K~ 3 effects on growth of rat glioma and human glioblastoma multiforme cells in vitro." *Acta neurologica belgica* 104 (2004): 106–110.

16) Kawakita, Hideaki, et al. "Growth inhibitory effects of vitamin K2 on colon cancer cell lines via different types of cell death including autophagy and apoptosis." *International journal of molecular medicine* 23.6 (2009): 709–716.

17) Yoshida, Tsuyoshi, et al. "Apoptosis induction of vitamin K2 in lung carcinoma cell lines: the possibility of vitamin K2 therapy for lung cancer." *International journal of oncology* 23.3 (2003): 627–632.

18) Showalter, Shayna L., et al. "Naturally occurring K vitamins inhibit pancreatic cancer cell survival through a caspase-dependent pathway." *Journal of gastroenterology and hepatology* 25.4 (2010): 738–744.

19) Ogawa, Mutsumi, et al. "Vitamins K2, K3 and K5 exert antitumor effects on established colorectal cancer in mice by inducing apoptotic death of tumor cells." *International journal of oncology* 31.2 (2007): 323–331.

20) Jiang, Yu, et al. "Vitamin K4 induces tumor cytotoxicity in human prostate carcinoma PC-3 cells via the mitochondria-related apoptotic pathway." *Die Pharmazie-An International Journal of Pharmaceutical Sciences* 68.6 (2013): 442–448.

21) *Vitamin K: The Forgotten Vitamin.* by Patrick Holford, Jul 2012.

22) Okamoto, Hiroshi. "Vitamin K and rheumatoid arthritis." IUBMB life 60.6 (2008): 355–361.

23) Seyama, et al. "Comparative effects of vitamin K2 and vitamin E on experimental arteriosclerosis." *International journal for vitamin and nutrition research* 69.1 (1999): 23–26.

24) Pizzorno, L. "Vitamin K2: Optimal levels essential for the prevention of age-associated chronic disease. Longevity Medicine Review Web site." (2015).

25) Knapen, M. H. J., L. J. Schurgers, and C. Vermeer. "Vitamin K2 supplementation improves hip bone geometry and bone strength indices in postmenopausal women." *Osteoporosis international* 18.7 (2007): 963–972.

26) Pearson, Debra A. "Bone health and osteoporosis: the role of vitamin K and potential antagonism by anticoagulants." *Nutrition in Clinical Practice* 22.5 (2007): 517–544.

27) Vitamin K – Linus Pauling Institute Oregon State U

28) The Remarkable Anticancer Properties of Vitamin K, by Felix DiFara *Life Extension Magazine.*

29) Nakaya, K., et al. "Vitamin K2 as a Chemotherapeutic Agent for Treating Ovarian Cancer." Ovarian Cancer-Clinical and Therapeutic Perspectives. *InTech*, 2012.

30) Plaza, Steven M. "The anticancer effects of vitamin K." Alternative Medicine Review 8.3 (2003): 303–318. Anticancer Effects of vitamin K Plaza Steven .*Alt Med Review* 2003

31) Karasawa, Satoki, et al. "Vitamin K2 covalently binds to Bak and induces Bak-mediated apoptosis." Molecular pharmacology 83.3 (2013): 613–620. Mol Pharmacol. 2013 Mar;83(3):613–20.

32) Yokoyama, Tomohisa, et al. "Vitamin K2 induces autophagy and apoptosis simultaneously in leukemia cells." *Autophagy* 4.5 (2008): 629–640.

33) Shibayama-Imazu, Toshiko, et al. "Production of superoxide and dissipation of mitochondrial transmembrane potential by vitamin K2 trigger apoptosis in human ovarian cancer TYK-nu cells." *Apoptosis* 11.9 (2006): 1535–1543.

34) Shibayama-Imazu, Toshiko, Toshihiro Aiuchi, and Kazuyasu Nakaya. "Vitamin K2-mediated apoptosis in cancer cells: Role of mitochondrial transmembrane potential." *Vitamins & Hormones* 78 (2008): 211–226.

35) Nakaya, K., et al. Vitamin K2 as a Chemotherapeutic Agent for Treating Ovarian Cancer. *INTECH Open Access Publisher*, 2012.

36) Kiely, Maeve, et al. "Real-time cell analysis of the inhibitory effect of vitamin K2 on adhesion and proliferation of breast cancer cells." *Nutrition Research* 35.8 (2015): 736–743.

37) Theuwissen, Elke, Egbert Smit, and Cees Vermeer. "The role of vitamin K in soft-tissue calcification." *Advances in Nutrition: An International Review Journal* 3.2 (2012): 166–173.

38) Masuda, Yutaka, et al. "Geranylgeraniol potently induces caspase-3-like activity during apoptosis in human leukemia U937 cells." *Biochemical and biophysical research communications* 234.3 (1997): 641–645.

39) Viana, S. Mejia. "Non Typical Risk Factors in Atherosclerosis and Coronary Disease. It Is Time to Open the Box and Look Outside." *J Clin Trials Cardiol* 4.1 (2017): 1–5.

40) Zheng, Shuan, Zhangsuo Liu, and Donghai Wang. "The efficacy of vitamin K on vascular calcification for chronic renal failure patient receiving dialysis." *Int J Clin Exp Med* 9.9 (2016): 18092–18097.

41) Scheiber, Daniel, et al. "High-dose menaquinone-7 supplementation reduces cardiovascular calcification in a murine model of extraosseous calcification." *Nutrients* 7.8 (2015): 6991–7011.

43) Shea, M. Kyla, et al. "Vitamin K supplementation and progression of coronary artery calcium in older men and women–." *The American journal of clinical nutrition* 89.6 (2009): 1799–1807.

44) van den Heuvel, Ellen GHM, et al. "Circulating uncarboxylated matrix Gla protein, a marker of vitamin K status, as a risk factor of cardiovascular disease." *Maturitas* 77.2 (2014): 137–141.

45) Mayer, Otto, et al. "Desphospho-uncarboxylated matrix Gla-protein is associated with mortality risk in patients with chronic stable vascular disease." *Atherosclerosis* 235.1 (2014): 162–168.

46) Merkel, Richard L. "The use of menadione bisulfite and ascorbic acid in the treatment of nausea and vomiting of pregnancy." *American Journal of Obstetrics & Gynecology* 64.2 (1952): 416–418.

47) Takami, Akiyoshi, et al. "Successful therapy of myelodysplastic syndrome with menatetrenone, a vitamin K2 analog." International journal of hematology 69.1 (1999): 24-26.

Linus Pauling: Heart-Disease Prevention with Vitamin C

I ONCE HAD A CONVERSATION with a cardiologist friend of mine. I casually mentioned the Linus Pauling Theory of heart disease, the idea that vitamin C and a few amino acids could prevent and reverse heart disease. The response from my cardiologist friend was hearty laughter that anyone would suggest such nonsense. "Surely," he asked, "you must be joking?"

My cardiologist friend and the rest of the mainstream medical system have no clue about the steamroller coming to health care, aiming right at the huge profits from diagnosis and treatment of heart disease, a multi-billion dollar industry in the U.S. The cardiac cath lab and cardiac bypass surgery program will be flattened, the first casualties of the Internet medical information revolution providing consumers with knowledge about a safe and cheap supplement program to reverse heart disease, the Linus Pauling Protocol. The time has come for the old dinosaurs to go. In the near future, thanks to Linus Pauling, heart disease will become a curiosity of the past, like the disappearance of gastric ulcers after the invention of antacids and antibiotics. (50–51)

The Linus Pauling Protocol: Vitamin C

Vitamin C is required to make a protein called collagen. Vitamin C deficiency is a disease called scurvy. Why is collagen so important? Collagen is the most abundant protein in the body. It is the structural protein used to make connective tissues, bones, teeth, hair, and arteries. Strong collagen is important for a strong body.

Vitamin C Deficiency Results in Poor Lysine Cross-linking on Collagen

How does vitamin C produce strong collagen? How does this work? Vitamin C is required for lysyl hydroxylase, an enzyme responsible for attaching the lysine residues together on adjacent collagen strands. Vitamin C deficiency results in weakened collagen strands caused by disrupted lysine cross-linking. The resulting weakened collagen results in a widespread problem in the connective tissues, bones, teeth, skin, hair, arteries, etc.

Steps in Collagen Synthesis

How are the fibrils crosslinked? This is done by combining two lysine molecules with the help of the enzyme lysine hydroxylase, which requires vitamin C. Lack of vitamin C results in poor collagen cross-linking. In the full-blown vitamin C deficiency disease called scurvy, the structural elements of the body literally fall apart: collagen breaks down and is not replaced; the joints wear out, the small arteries begin to crack and degenerate, the skin shows easy bruising and bleeding as small vessels rupture throughout the body, and the teeth may loosen and fall out.

Linus Pauling: Heart Disease Is a Chronic Scurvy Condition

Linus Pauling was unquestionably the greatest scientist of the twentieth century. All of modern biochemistry and molecular biology chemistry are based on Pauling's work, especially his discovery and elucidation of the chemical bond. Pauling is the only scientist to be awarded two unshared Nobel prizes.

Pauling's later years were devoted to heart disease. In 1989, he published with Dr. Matthias Rath "A Unified Theory of Human Cardiovascular Disease," in which he states that atherosclerotic plaques in heart disease are actually part of process of repairing the arterial damage caused by chronic vitamin C deficiency. (13)(26,27)

In essence, Pauling said that heart disease is a manifestation of chronic scurvy, and atherosclerotic plaque is a mechanism that evolved to repair or patch blood vessels and arteries damaged because of a lack of vitamin C. Pauling also said that atherosclerotic plaque formation can be prevented or reversed with vitamin C, lysine, and proline. These are nutritional supplements available at any health food store for a few dollars.

Atherosclerotic Plaques

Plaque deposits found in human aortas are made up of a form of cholesterol called lipoprotein (a) also called lipoprotein little a, or Lp(a). These plaques are not randomly distributed throughout the arterial tree; rather, their distribution is restricted to sites of high mechanical stress, such as bifurcations (places where an artery branches out), and areas of motion such as the surface of the heart (coronary arteries). In the early 1950s, a Canadian, G. C. Willis, MD, made these same observations, and they have been confirmed by 60 years of coronary and peripheral arteriography at major medical centers. (1–4)

Imagine stepping on your garden hose a thousand times a day. You will soon notice cracks in the wall of the garden hose. This is the same process that happens in the artery. As these cracks open up, the collagen strands in the wall of the artery are teased apart. The triple helix collagen strands that are normally bound together with lysine crosslinks are now separated and exposed to the circulating bloodstream.

The lysine residues look like little flags waving from the damaged collagen strand. The exposed lysine strands are available for binding to circulating lipoprotein (a), which is a special form of cholesterol that has lysine receptors and is known to increase heart-disease risk. This attachment of lipoprotein(a) to the free lysine residues of damaged collagen initiates the atherosclerotic process. Over time, this process builds larger plaque deposits, which eventually narrow the inner diameter of the artery, causing a blockage or leading to plaque rupture and thrombosis, a catastrophic event that may cause heart attack or sudden death.

Experiments done in 1997 by Dr. Nataya Boonmark on genetically modified mice that have "knocked out" the lysine binding sites on lipoprotein (a) show a fivefold reduction in atherosclerotic plaque formation. (17)

Can You Make Vitamin C? No, You Can't

We humans cannot make vitamin C in our liver, as all other animals do. Fifty million years ago, a genetic mutation in our ancestors "knocked out" the final enzyme in the hepatic synthesis of vitamin C. The missing enzyme is called GLO (gulano lactone oxidase). (42–43) Primates such as gorillas, chimpanzees, and orangutans also share this same GLO mutation and cannot make vitamin C. In addition, all primates share with humans a susceptibility to heart disease. (45–47)

Almost All Animals Can Make Vitamin C, but the Guinea Pig Can't

Except for humans and primates, all animals have the three enzymes in the liver that can synthesize vitamin C from glucose (a simple sugar). One major exception is the guinea pig, which is really a rodent and not a pig. The guinea pig, for some unexplained reason, shares with humans the identical GLO genetic mutation and also lacks the GLO enzyme, just as we do. (43) This makes the guinea pig an ideal experimental model for human diseases. By the way, although animals that make vitamin C never get heart disease, the guinea pig, which lacks the ability to synthesize vitamin C, also gets heart disease.

Note: I am referring to atherosclerotic vascular heart disease in animals. Dogs and Cats DO succumb to other common types of heart disease such as cardiomyopathy and heart worm etc.)

Animals that don't make vitamin C do get atherosclerotic heart disease. This should be starting to become clear now.

Animal Scientific Support for the Pauling Unified Theory

As mentioned above, guinea pigs are especially well suited for studies of atherosclerosis because they are unable to make their own vitamin C, and in addition, they develop atherosclerotic plaques similar to those found in humans.

G. C. Willis, a Canadian doctor, conducted research on guinea pigs in the 1950s showing that, when deprived of dietary vitamin, C they developed atherosclerotic plaques, while guinea pigs who were given plentiful vitamin C were protected. In addition, guinea pigs fed a vitamin-C-deficient diet had elevated lipoprotein (a) levels along with the increased plaque in the arteries. (1–4)

Similar findings were demonstrated by Dr. Nobuyo Maeda in 2000 in genetically engineered mice lacking the GLO enzyme. The GLO-deficient mice fed a vitamin-C-deficient diet developed atherosclerotic plaques in the aorta with characteristic deranged collagen cross-linking. GLO-deficient mice fed vitamin C were protected. (18)

Human Studies Supporting the Linus Pauling Theory

Optometrist Dr. Sydney Bush's retinal artery observations support the Pauling theory. Using modern equipment to non-invasively photograph the retinal arteries of the eye before and after vitamin C supplementation in humans, Dr. Bush has documented the reversal of atherosclerotic plaque with vitamin C supplementation. Unfortunately, Dr. Sidney Bush's discoveries were not well received. His optometry license was revoked in 1993. (19) (39–40)

Why has no drug company sponsored a double-blind placebo-controlled study of Vitamin C? Vitamin C is a natural substance which cannot be patented. Since there are no patents and no drugs involved, no drug company would ever invest the 250 million dollars to fund such a study with no potential for financial return.

The Physician's Health Study—Don't Waste Your Money On Vitamins!!

Using public funds, the NIH funded a large study called The Physicians' Health Study II, which evaluated Vitamins C and E in heart disease. An article by Howard D. Sesso et al. reporting on this study was published Nov. 9, 2008 in *JAMA*. (21) The study found that vitamin C and E did not prevent mortality from heart disease, results that are completely opposite to massive previously published research and anecdotal case reports.

However, a closer look shows a few glaring errors in study design. The dosage of vitamin C was set too low, at one-tenth the dosage recommended by the Linus Pauling protocol, and lysine was not provided. While the Sesso study showed no mortality benefit, many previous studies, such as the Enstrom Study, showed a striking 40% reduction in all-cause mortality over 6 years from the same 500 mg daily vitamin C dosage.(23) The Paul Knekt study showed a 25% reduction in heart disease risk with daily 700 mg vitamin C.(24) Two previous studies from Japan and Finland showed that vitamin C reduces risk for stroke, another form of atherosclerotic disease.(52-53) There are many more like these.

Since favorable results would be financially destructive to the drug and hospital industries, a cynic might suggest that vested interests at work in the Sesso study intended to discredit vitamin C, as corporate influence in medical research has been documented many times in the past. (21) It is not difficult to design a medical study to fail. I regard this as merely another example of the information war waged by corporate mainstream medicine against natural medicine.

Enstrom Study: 500 mg Vitamin C Reduces Mortality 40% over 6 years

Enstrom showed that increasing vitamin C intake had a dramatic 40% reduction in mortality benefit, which exceeds any statin drug study ever conducted. (23)

Linus Pauling Protocol for Prevention and Reversal of Plaque

If heart disease is chronic scurvy, caused by chronic vitamin C deficiency, then it makes sense to supplement with vitamin C in the amounts needed to make strong collagen and prevent arterial damage from mechanical stress.

Pauling devised a clever yet simple method to address the issue of lipo-protein (a) attaching to the lysine residues on the damaged collagen fibers in the arterial wall. He recommended supplementing with 2–4 grams of lysine per day. The additional lysine in the bloodstream attaches to the receptor sites on the lipoprotein (a) molecules, preventing attachment to the arterial wall. This prevents the initiation of the atherosclerotic process. In addition, vitamin C and lysine are both important precursors for building strong collagen, which makes strong arteries. Along with Lysine, some of the collagen cross-linking is done with another amino acid called proline, which was also added to the treatment protocol.

Linus Pauling Protocol Validated with Calcium Score

In 1996, a CAT-scan coronary-calcium-score study of 55 patients vali-dated the Linus Pauling protocol. (14) For patients receiving the protocol plus additional minerals and cofactors, the annual progression of their calcium score was reduced to 15%, compared to 44% before the program started. (14) In 1994, a patent was issued for the Linus Pauling Protocol.

What Is the Linus Pauling Protocol?

- L-Ascorbate (vitamin C) 5–6 grams a day in divided doses
- L-Lysine 5 grams a day in divided doses
- L-Proline 2–3 grams a day in divided doses
- Tocotrienols vitamin E 200 mg /d

Additions to the protocol:

- MK-7 and MK-4 versions of vitamin K2
- Aged Garlic

These supplements can be obtained at any health food store as tablets or capsules for 40 to 150 dollars a month.

Vitamin E: Good or Bad, Yes or No, Blessing or Curse?

Steve Hickey and Hilary Roberts come right out on page 167 of their book on vitamin C and make the statement, *"Vitamin C and Tocotrienols can reverse coronary artery disease."* They would add the Tocotrienol form of vitamin E to the Linus Pauling Protocol. Regarding heart disease and atherosclerotic vascular disease, the authors state that *"on the available evidence, the combination of Vitamin C and Tocotrienols could be curative with no known harmful effects."*

Opposition to the Linus Pauling Protocol by Mainstream Medicine

If you are facing the prospect of a coronary artery bypass, you might ask the obvious question: *"Why hasn't my cardiologist told me about this information and started me on the Linus Pauling Protocol?"* Most cardiologists either don't know about it or ignore it because of the information war going on between mainstream medicine and natural medicine. Cardiologists read medical journals that regularly run incorrect and biased articles saying vitamin C is useless for prevention and reversal of heart disease, such as the 2008 Sesso study. (21)

Diagnosing and treating heart disease with expensive tests and procedures, such as coronary angiography, angioplasty, stenting, and bypass operation is the most profitable part of hospital big business. That's why hospitals compete and fight with each other over the rights to expand and build larger cardiac-catheterization labs and cardiac bypass operation programs. These programs are huge money makers for the national hospital system.

What would happen if there were a cheap and effective way to reverse and prevent heart disease, (e.g., the Linus Pauling Protocol)? Heart disease would become an uncommon illness. With fewer heart patients to treat, the multi-million dollar cardiac catheterization labs and cardiac bypass programs at your local hospital would become obsolete and disappear. This would be a financial catastrophe for mainstream medicine.

With so much money and vested interest at stake, you can imagine why it is not prudent for a cardiologist to bring up the benefits of the Linus Pauling Protocol in friendly conversation while lunching in the doctor's dining hall. That would be an instant ticket off the medical staff roster and out the hospital door, and the end of a lucrative cardiology practice. What cardiologist in their right mind would do that? It is easier for mainstream cardiologists to simply laugh it off as a joke and return to the routine in the cardiac catheter laboratory (cath lab).

Here is one final question about the Linus Pauling Protocol. If Linus Pauling were alive today, would he have incorporated the latest medical discovery that atherosclerotic plaque is infected biofilm? I believe so.

♦　♦　♦　♦　♦

♦ References for Chapter 10

1) Willis, G. C. "Intimal ground substance in atherosclerosis." *Canadian Medical Association Journal* 69.1 (1953): 17.

2) Willis, G. C., A. W. Light, and W. S. Gow. "Serial arteriography in atherosclerosis." *Canadian Medical Association Journal* 71.6 (1954): 562.

3) Willis, G. C., and S. Fishman. "Ascorbic acid content of human arterial tissue." *Canadian Medical Association Journal* 72.7 (1955): 500.

4) Willis, G. C. "The reversibility of atherosclerosis." *Canadian Medical Association Journal* 77.2 (1957): 106.

5) Paterson, J. C. "Capillary rupture with intimal hemorrhage in the causation of cerebral vascular lesions." *Arch Pathol* 29 (1940): 345–354.

6) J. C. "Some factors in the causation of intimal haemorrhages and in the precipitation of coronary thrombi." *Canadian Medical Association Journal* 44.2 (1941): 114.

7) Fernandez, Maria Luz, and Jeff S. Volek. "Guinea pigs: a suitable animal model to study lipoprotein metabolism, atherosclerosis and inflammation." *Nutrition & metabolism* 3.1 (2006): 17.

8) Fernandez, Maria Luz. "Guinea pigs as models for cholesterol and lipoprotein metabolism." *The Journal of nutrition* 131.1 (2001): 10–20.

9) FUJITANI, TAKAO, et al. "Experimental atherosclerosis with ascorbic acid deficiency." *Japanese circulation journal* 35.12 (1971): 1559–1565.

10) Rath, Matthias, and Linus Pauling. "Immunological evidence for the accumulation of lipoprotein (a) in the atherosclerotic lesion of the hypoascorbemic guinea pig." *Proceedings of the National Academy of Sciences* 87.23 (1990): 9388–9390.

11) Rath, Matthias, and Linus Pauling. "Hypothesis: lipoprotein (a) is a surrogate for ascorbate." *Proceedings of the National Academy of Sciences* 87.16 (1990): 6204–6207.

12) Pauling, Linus. "Case report: Lysine/ascorbate-related amelioration of angina pectoris." *J. Orthomolecular Med* 6 (1991): 144–146.

13) Rath, Matthias, and Linus Pauling. "A unified theory of human cardiovascular disease leading the way to the abolition of this disease as a cause for human mortality." *Journal of Orthomolecular Medicine* 7.1 (1992): 5–15.

14) Niedzwiecki, Aleksandra, and Matthias Rath. "Nutritional supplement program halts progression of early coronary atherosclerosis documented by ultrafast computed tomography." *Journal of Applied Nutrition* 48 (1996): 68–78.

15) Chakrabarty, Sunil, et al. "Protective role of ascorbic acid against lipid peroxidation and myocardial injury." *Molecular and cellular biochemistry* 111.1–2 (1992): 41–47.

16) Price, Kendall D., Catherine SC Price, and Robert D. Reynolds. "Hyperglycemia-induced ascorbic acid deficiency promotes endothelial dysfunction and the development of atherosclerosis." *Atherosclerosis* 158.1 (2001): 1–12.

17) Boonmark, Nataya W., et al. "Modification of apolipoprotein (a) lysine binding site reduces atherosclerosis in transgenic mice." *Journal of Clinical Investigation* 100.3 (1997): 558.

18) Maeda, Nobuyo, et al. "Aortic wall damage in mice unable to synthesize ascorbic acid." *Proceedings of the National Academy of Sciences* 97.2 (2000): 841–846.

19) Sidney Bush Presentation at 2003 medical meeting: sidney-j-bush-cardio-retinometry-vitamin-c-2013

20) Simon, Joel A., et al. "Relation of Ascorbic Acid to Coronary Artery Calcium The Coronary Artery Risk Development in Young Adults Study." *American journal of epidemiology* 159.6 (2004): 581–588.

21) Sesso, Howard D., et al. "Vitamins E and C in the prevention of cardiovascular disease in men: the Physicians' Health Study II randomized controlled trial." *Jama* 300.18 (2008): 2123–2133.

22) Libby, Peter, and Masanori Aikawa. "Vitamin C, collagen, and cracks in the plaque." (2002): 1396–1398.

23) Enstrom, James E., Linda E. Kanim, and Morton A. Klein. "Vitamin C intake and mortality among a sample of the United States population." *Epidemiology* (1992): 194–202.

24) Knekt, Paul, et al. "Antioxidant vitamins and coronary heart disease risk: a pooled analysis of nine cohorts." The American Journal of Clinical Nutrition 80.6 (2004): 1508–1520.

25) Hampl, Jeffrey S., Christopher A. Taylor, and Carol S. Johnston. "Vitamin C deficiency and depletion in the United States: the third national health and nutrition examination survey, 1988 to 1994." American journal of public health 94.5 (2004): 870–875.

26) The Unified Theory, The Long Neglected Theory of Cardiovascular and Heart Disease By Owen Richard Fonorow 2002

27) English, Jim, and Hyla Cass. "Linus Pauling Unified Theory of Human Cardiovascular Disease: The Collagen Connection." Nutrition Review 2013.

28) Peltier, Marcel, et al. "Elevated serum lipoprotein (a) level is an independent marker of severity of thoracic aortic atherosclerosis." Chest 121.5 (2002): 1589–1594.

29) Reblin, Tjark, et al. "Extraction of lipoprotein (a), apo B, and apo E from fresh human arterial wall and atherosclerotic plaques." Atherosclerosis 113.2 (1995): 179–188.

30) Pepin, Judith M., June A. O'neil, and Henry F. Hoff. "Quantification of apo [a] and apoB in human atherosclerotic lesions." Journal of lipid research 32.2 (1991): 317–327.

31) Hughes, Steven D., et al. "Lipoprotein (a) vascular accumulation in mice. In vivo analysis of the role of lysine binding sites using recombinant adenovirus." The Journal of clinical investigation 100.6 (1997): 1493–1500.

32) Yamauchi, Mitsuo, and Masashi Shiiba. "Lysine hydroxylation and cross-linking of collagen." Post-translational Modifications of Proteins. Humana Press, 2008. 95–108.

33) Frei, Balz, Laura England, and Bruce N. Ames. "Ascorbate is an outstanding antioxidant in human blood plasma." Proceedings of the National Academy of Sciences 86.16 (1989): 6377–6381.

34) Ohta, Yuriko, and Morimitsu Nishikimi. "Random nucleotide substitutions in primate nonfunctional gene for L-gulono-γ-lactone oxidase, the missing enzyme in L-ascorbic acid biosynthesis." Biochimica et Biophysica Acta (BBA)-General Subjects 1472.1–2 (1999): 408–411.

36) Pinnell, SHELDON R. "Regulation of collagen biosynthesis by ascorbic acid: a review." *The Yale journal of biology and medicine* 58.6 (1985): 553.

37) same as 17) Boonmark, Nataya W., et al. "Modification of apolipoprotein (a) lysine binding site reduces atherosclerosis in transgenic mice." The Journal of clinical investigation 100.3 (1997): 558–564.

38) Person, Margaret M. Characterization and Quantification of Myocardial Collagen in the Borderline Hypertensive Rat. Diss. Youngstown State University, 2007.

39) Bush S. J. Cardioretinometry Rapid Response BMJ 23rd July

40) Bush S. J. "Emperor's New Clothes?" *Rapid Response BMJ* 25th Nov. 2004.

41) Wong TY et al. Prospective cohort study of retinal vessel diameters and risk of hypertension. BMJ 2004 329:79 (10th July) pub 2nd Jne.

42) Inai Y et al. (2003), "The Whole Structure of the Human Non-Functional L-Guluno-gamma-Lactone Oxidase Gene – the Gene Responsible for Scurvy – and the Evolution of Repetitive Sequences Thereon," *J Nutr Sci Vitaminology* 49:315–319.

43) Nishikimi, M., Toshihide Kawai, and Kunio Yagi. "Guinea pigs possess a highly mutated gene for L-gulono-gamma-lactone oxidase, the key enzyme for L-ascorbic acid biosynthesis missing in this species." *Journal of Biological Chemistry* 267.30 (1992): 21967–21972.

44) Centers for Disease Control and Prevention (CDC. "Decline in deaths from heart disease and stroke—United States, 1900–1999." MMWR. *Morbidity and mortality weekly report* 48.30 (1999): 649.

45) Nishikimi, M., et al. "Cloning and chromosomal mapping of the human nonfunctional gene for L-gulono-gamma-lactone oxidase, the enzyme for L-ascorbic acid biosynthesis missing in man." *Journal of Biological Chemistry* 269.18 (1994): 13685–13688.

46) Maeda, Nobuyo, et al. "Aortic wall damage in mice unable to synthesize ascorbic acid." *Proceedings of the National Academy of Sciences* 97.2 (2000): 841–846.

47) Nishikimi, Morimitsu, and Kunio Yagi. "Molecular basis for the deficiency in humans of gulonolactone oxidase, a key enzyme for ascorbic acid biosynthesis." *The American journal of clinical nutrition* 54.6 (1991): 1203S-1208S.

48) Deruelle, Fabien, and Bertrand Baron. "Vitamin C: is supplementation necessary for optimal health?." *The Journal of Alternative and Complementary Medicine* 14.10 (2008): 1291–1298.

50) Ritterman, Jeffrey B. "To Err is Human: Can American Medicine Learn from Past Mistakes?." *The Permanente journal* 21 (2017).

51) Ahmed, Niyaz. "23 years of the discovery of Helicobacter pylori: Is the debate over?." (2005): 17

52) Yokoyama, Tetsuji, et al. "Serum vitamin C concentration was inversely associated with subsequent 20-year incidence of stroke in a Japanese rural community: the Shibata study." Stroke 31.10 (2000): 2287-2294.

53) Kurl, S., et al. "Plasma vitamin C modifies the association between hypertension and risk of stroke." stroke 33.6 (2002): 1568-1573.

Vitamin E, Heart Disease, and Tocotrienols

YEARS AGO, THE FAMILY ENJOYED a rafting vacation on the Snake River in Idaho. Everyone survived the river adventure, and we later explored the little town of Coeur D'Alene with its second-hand bookstore called the Bookworm. At the store, I picked up an old (1964) copy of *Vitamin E: Your Key to a Healthy Heart*, by Herbert Baily. I later learned the book had sold a million copies and stimulated considerable interest in vitamin E. It was one of the first books to make vitamins popular.

Vitamin E Discovered in 1922

In 1922, an obscure researcher named Herbert McLean Evans discovered Vitamin E. The chemical structure was determined in 1938, and Evans named it from the Greek word *tocopherol*, meaning "to bear young," since it seemed to be associated with fertility. In the 1930s and 1940s, two Canadian cardiologists, Wilfred and Evan Shute, treated 30,000 patients with natural vitamin E and reported considerable success in reversing heart disease.

Doubts About Vitamin E: "Vitamin E Is Deadly!!"

You may have seen news reports that Vitamin E is dangerous, deadly, and increases mortality. These media stories were based on an article by Edgar Miller in the 2005 *Annals of Internal Medicine,* a meta-analysis of 19 studies on Vitamin E, concluding that Vitamin E increases mortality. One of these media stories, "High Dose of Vitamin E Increases Death Risk," by Steve

Sternberg, in *USA Today*, reported the following:

High-dose vitamin E supplements taken daily can increase a person's risk of premature death, researchers said Wednesday. People who take daily doses of 400 international units or higher are about 10% more likely to die of a variety of causes than people who take smaller doses or no vitamin E, according to an analysis of 14 studies conducted between 1993 and 2004. Many of the studies did not specify causes of death, but researchers believe patients died of all the usual causes, including heart disease and cancer. (2)

The effect of Miller's Vitamin E article was that many people stopped using vitamin E. An excellent rebuttal to Miller by Dr. Mark Houston pointed out the type of vitamin E used in Miller's meta-analysis was synthetic dl alpha-tocopherol. Dr. Houston says:

None of the 19 studies in Miller's review article included any of the other seven forms of vitamin E, and in fact, most of them used the synthetic d, l alpha-tocopherol form. It is important to distinguish natural vitamin E from the synthetic Vitamin E which is to be avoided. (15)

Amazingly, another negative Vitamin E study published by Sesso in *JAMA* Nov 9, 2008 again used the synthetic form of Vitamin E. (9) You would think that doctors would be intelligent enough to use the natural form of vitamin E.

Here is another disturbing fact: Dr. Sesso's negative vitamin E study was sponsored by Wyeth, a drug company with a long history of animosity to natural treatments. The paper also disclosed that many of the authors received funds from Wyeth, Merck, Bristol-Meyers Squibb, Astra Zeneca, Pfizer, and Bayer.

The Different Types of Vitamin E: Synthetic vs. Natural

Natural vitamin E is in the "D" form (meaning dextro, which is Latin for "right-handed"). Synthetic vitamin E is a combination of the D and L form (i.e., DL). The synthetic form is cheaper but is not recommended. There are eight types of tocopherols in nature including, the alpha, delta, gamma forms.

Evidence that the Natural Form of Vitamin E Is Beneficial

Two landmark vitamin E studies were published in 1993 in the *New England Journal of Medicine*. Dr. Eric Rimm's study showed a 36% reduction in heart disease in men taking the relatively modest 60 IU vitamin E daily in the diet. (49) Meir Stamfer's study showed a 33% reduction in heart attacks in women with the highest dietary vitamin E consumption. (50)

More Studies Showing Benefits of Natural Vitamin E

In 1992, Verlangeri published a study in which natural vitamin E reversed atherosclerosis in a primate model. (27) A 1995 study published in *JAMA* by Howard N. Hodis showed that Vitamin E caused regression of atherosclerosis on serial coronary angiography. Hodis concluded:

These results indicate an association between supplementary vitamin E intake and angiographically demonstrated reduction in coronary artery lesion progression. (28)(44)

In 1996, Stephens published his study in *Lancet* showing that tocopherol (vitamin E) given to patients with advanced coronary artery disease reduced the risk of non-fatal MI by 77% (but did not decrease total mortality in this study). (45)

In 2000, Boaz published a study in Lancet showing that 800 IU/daily of natural Vitamin E reduced heart attacks by 70% over 1.4 years in hemodialysis patients. (53)

Reversing Carotid Stenosis with Natural Vitamin E

In 1997, D. K. Kooyenga and Marvin Bierenbaum presented their data on reversal of atherosclerosis in carotid stenosis with mixed tocopherols and tocotrienols at a meeting in Montreal. (30)(33)

The Bierenbaum study was done at the Kenneth Jordan Heart Research Foundation in New Jersey. The five-year study evaluated 50 patients who had stenosis of the carotid artery. One group of 25 patients received 650 mgs of tocotrienols plus tocopherols. The other group of 25 received a placebo. All patients had serial carotid sonography every six months. In the placebo group, 15 patients showed worsening of the stenosis, eight remained stable, and two showed some improvement. In the Tocotrienol (plus tocopherol) group, three patients showed minor worsening, and 12 remained stable. Ten patients showed regression of stenosis with improvement.

The 21st Century Form of Vitamin E – Tocotrienol

Not only is there a difference between synthetic and natural vitamin E, there is also a new form of vitamin E called tocotrienol, the more biologically useful form. What is the difference between the tocopherol and tocotrienol?

Tocopherol Straight Tail, Tocotrienol Curved Tail

Tocotrienol is identical to tocopherol except for the three double bonds in the tail portion. These three double bonds create a kinked configuration of the "tail" that allows the molecule more mobility through lipid membranes. The three double bonds represent an "unsaturated" side chain which allows the molecule to penetrate into saturated lipid membrane layers in various target organs. The double bond also indicates a state of electron desaturation, meaning that it can accept electrons readily as an antioxidant. Thus, the tocotrienol form is superior to tocopherol as an antioxidant, serving to reverse lipid peroxidation.

About 99% of medical research since the discovery of Vitamin E has been devoted to the tocopherol form, and 1% on the tocotrienol form. This seems to be changing. There are no synthetic forms of tocotrienols available, only natural ones.

Processed Trans-Fats vs. Natural Oils

Remember the difference between processed trans-fats and natural oils, such as cold-pressed olive oil? The unhealthy trans fats have a straight carbon tail, because they have been processed, so the carbons are located on the opposite sides of the double bonds (trans). The healthy natural oils have a curved configuration of the carbon tail because the carbons are on the same side (cis) of the double bond. This difference is called cis-trans isomerism.

Oleic acid is a cis-unsaturated fatty acid that comprises 55–80% of cold-pressed olive oil.

Curved Tail in Tocotrienols

Similar to natural oils, the beneficial tocotrienols have a curved carbon tail, giving it more biological activity than its tocopherol counterpart. Note that the tail is not stationary but actually vibrates back and forth in space like a pendulum, absorbing energy within the membrane bi-layer. Although in the case of tocotrienols the three double bonds are in the trans-configuration, this is sufficient to bend the tail configuration significantly.

Health Benefits of Tocotrienol Form of Vitamin E

Tocotrienols are protective in stroke-induced injuries. Natural palm tocotrienol complex fed to hypertensive rats led to increased tocotrienols level in the brain, and more protection against stroke-induced injury compared to controls. (42).

Tocotrienol reversed atherosclerosis in carotid artery stenosis in human study by Watkins and Bierenbaum. (39)

Tocotrienols and cholesterol reduction: Gamma tocotrienol inhibit hepatic cholesterol synthesis without interfering with CoQ10 production, thus reducing LDL cholesterol levels safely. (7)

ApoE Mouse Studies Show Tocotrienol Protective

The ApoE Mouse Model is a genetically modified mouse that develops atherosclerosis of the aorta. Two separate studies, by Qureshi and by Black, showed that feeding Tocotrienols to the ApoE mice virtually eliminates atherosclerotic plaque. (46–47) Tocotrienols reduced the atherosclerosis plaque **by 98%,** an amazing result. On the other hand, Tocopherols had no such beneficial effect in ApoE mice in the study by Shaish (1999), who found no change in plaque size with Tocopherols. (48)

Dr. Barrie Tan discovered a plant in South America called annatto (or bixin) which provides pure tocotrienols. Dr. Tan owns the patent on the extraction process. (7)

Reversing Coronary Artery Disease

Chapter 10 discussed the use of high-dose vitamin C and the amino acid lysine, (the Linus Pauling Protocol) for reversing heart disease. Steve Hickey and Hilary Roberts state on page 167 of their book that *"vitamin C and Tocotrienols can reverse coronary artery disease."* (51) They would improve the Linus Pauling Protocol by adding the tocotrienol form of Vitamin E. Regarding heart disease, and atherosclerotic vascular disease, the authors state that *"on the available evidence, the combination of Vitamin C and Tocotrienols could be curative with no known harmful effects."* (51)

Future Research for the NIH, the Guinea Pig Model

Tocotrienols clearly prevent atherosclerosis in the ApoE mouse model. Further research in the guinea pig model should be done. Willis showed that vitamin-C-deprived guinea pigs develop atherosclerotic vascular disease. What if vitamin-C-deprived guinea pigs were given tocotrienols? I would predict tocotrienols would be beneficial, reducing or preventing atherosclerotic plaque formation. We await the outcomes of these and other studies.

The War on Heart Disease Is Over: We Won

Knowing the above, death from heart attack is both unnecessary and tragic. Information is now readily available explaining how heart disease can be prevented and reversed with simple inexpensive nutritional supplements at home. One need only read the information, and the evidence is overwhelming. There is no need for expensive drugs, cardiac-catheterization labs, or bypass operations. A simple combination of vitamin C, lysine, and the tocotrienol form of Vitamin E is sufficient to prevent and reverse heart disease.

Vitamin E : Bleeding Precautions:

Vitamin E can have a blood-thinning effect, so most surgeons and anesthesiologists will ask about vitamin E use prior to elective surgery, and request that the vitamin E be discontinued a week in advance of elective surgery to avoid bleeding complications.

♦　♦　♦　♦　♦

♦ References for Chapter 11

1) High dose vitamin E death warning, Thursday, 11 November, 2004. BBC News U.K.

2) Study: High dose of Vitamin E increases death risk By Steve Sternberg, *USA TODAY* 11/10/2004 6:50 PM

3–6) deleted

7) Tan, Barrie. "Vitamin E: Tocotrienols." (2012).

8) Sen, Chandan K., Savita Khanna, and Sashwati Roy. "Tocotrienols in health and disease: the other half of the natural vitamin E family." *Molecular aspects of medicine* 28.5–6 (2007): 692–728.

9) Howard D., et al. "Vitamins E and C in the prevention of cardiovascular disease in men: the Physicians' Health Study II randomized controlled trial." Jama 300.18 (2008): 2123–2133.

10) Designed To Fail: A Trial Without Meaning. Steve Hickey, Ph.D.; Damien Downing, M.B.B.S.; and Robert Verkerk, Ph.D., *Alliance for Natural Health.*

11) Devaraj, Sridevi, and Ishwarlal Jialal. "Failure of Vitamin E in Clinical Trials: Is Gamma-Tocopherol the Answer?." *Nutrition reviews* 63.8 (2005): 290–293.

12) Greenberg, E. Robert. "Vitamin E supplements: good in theory, but is the theory good?" *Annals of internal medicine* 142.1 (2005): 75–76.

13) Miller, Edgar R., et al. "Meta-analysis: high-dosage vitamin E supplementation may increase all-cause mortality." *Annals of internal medicine* 142.1 (2005): 37–46.

14) Guallar, Eliseo, Daniel F. Hanley, and Edgar R. Miller. "An editorial update: annus horribilis for vitamin E." *Annals of internal medicine* 143.2 (2005): 143–145.

15) Houston, Mark. "Meta-analysis, metaphysics and mythology-scientific and clinical perspective on the controversies regarding vitamin E for the prevention and treatment of disease in humans." *JANA* 8.1 (2005): 4–7.

16) Nesaretnam K, Ambra R, Selvaduray KR, et al. (2004). Tocotrienol-rich fraction from palm oil and gene expression in human breast cancer cells. *Annals of the New York Academy of Sciences* 1031: 143–157.

17) Conte C, Floridi A, Aisa C, et al. (2004). Gamma-Tocotrienol metabolism and antiproliferative effect in prostate cancer cells. *Annals of the New York Academy of Sciences* 1031: 391–394.

18) Hasselwander O, Kramer K, Hoppe PP, et al. (2002). Effects of feeding various tocotrienol sources on plasma lipids and aortic atherosclerotic lesions in cholesterol-fed rabbits. *FOOD RESEARCH INTERNATIONAL* 35 (2–3): 245–251

19) Montonen J, Knekt P, Jarvinen R, et al. (2004). Dietary antioxidant intake and risk of type 2 diabetes. *DIABETES CARE* 27 (2): 362–366.

20) Kappus H, Diplock AT. Tolerance and safety of vitamin E: a toxicological position report. *Free Radic Biol Med* 1992;13:55–'D074.

21) Hathcock, John N., et al. "Vitamins E and C are safe across a broad range of intakes." *The American journal of clinical nutrition* 81.4 (2005): 736–745.

22) Theriault, Andre, et al. "Tocotrienol: a review of its therapeutic potential." *Clinical biochemistry* 32.5 (1999): 309–319.

23) Sen, Chandan K., Savita Khanna, and Sashwati Roy. "Tocotrienol: the natural vitamin E to defend the nervous system?." *Annals of the New York Academy of Sciences* 1031.1 (2004): 127–142.

24) Das, Samarjit, et al. "Cardioprotection with palm tocotrienol: antioxidant activity of tocotrienol is linked with its ability to stabilize proteasomes." *American Journal of Physiology-Heart and Circulatory Physiology* 289.1 (2005): H361-H367.

25) Reversing Arteriosclerosis with Tocotrienols: An interview with Marvin Bierenbaum, MD and Tom Watkins, Ph.D. by Richard A. Passwater, Ph.D.

26) Passwater, R.A. (1992) Reversing atherosclerosis: An interview with Dr. Anthony Verlangieri. *Whole Foods* 15(9):27–30.

27) Verlangieri, A.J. and Bush, M.K. (1992) Effects of d-alpha-tocopherol supplementation on experimentally induced primate atherosclerosis. *J. Amer. Coll. Nutr.* 11:131–138.

28) Hodis, H.N.; Mack, W.J.; LaBree, L.; Cashin-Hemphill, L.; Sevanian, A.; Johnson, R. and Azen, S.P. (1995) Serial coronary angiographic evidence that antioxidant vitamin intake reduces progression of coronary artery atherosclerosis. *JAMA* 273(23):1849–1854.

29) Niedzwiecki, Aleksandra, and Matthias Rath. "Nutritional supplement program halts progression of early coronary atherosclerosis documented by ultrafast computed tomography." *Journal of Applied Nutrition* 48 (1996): 68–78.

30) Kooyenga, D.K.; Geller,M.; Watkins, T.R. and Bierenbaum, M.L. (July 29, 1997) Antioxidant-induced regression of carotid stenosis over three-years. Proceedings of the 16th International Congress of Nutrition. Montreal.

31) Fleischman, Alan I., Thomas Hayton, and M. L. Bierenbaum. "Serum lipids and certain dietary factors in young men with coronary heart disease." *Journal of the American Dietetic Association* 50 (1967): 112–115.

32) Bierenbaum, M.L.; Fleischman, A.I.; Raichelson, R.I.; Hayton, T. and Watson, P.B. (1973) Ten-year experience of modified-fat diets on younger men with coronary heart disease. *Lancet* 1 817:1404–1407.

33) Kooyenga, D. K., et al. "Palm oil antioxidant effects in patients with hyperlipidaemia and carotid stenosis-2 year experience." *Asia Pac J Clin Nutr* 6.1 (1997): 72–75.

34) Watkins, T.; Lenz, P.; Gapor, A.; Struck, M.: Tomeo, A. and Bierenbaum, M. (1993) Gamma- tocotrienol as a hypocholesterolemic and antioxidant agent in rats fed atherogenic diets. *Lipids* 28(12):1113–1118.

35) Suzuki, Y.J.; Tsuchiya, M.; Wassall, S.R.; Choo, Y.M.; Govil, G.; Kagan, V.E. and Packer, L. (1993) Structural and dynamic membrane properties of alpha-tocopherol and alpha-tocotrienol: implication to the molecular mechanism of their antioxidant potency. *Biochem.* 32:10692–10699.

36) Tomeo, A. C., et al. "Antioxidant effects of tocotrienols in patients with hyperlipidemia and carotid stenosis." *Lipids* 30.12 (1995): 1179–1183.

37) Serbinova, E. and Packer, L. (1994) Antioxidant and biological activities of palm oil vitamin E. *Food and Nutrition Bull.* 15:138–143.

38) Papas, Andreas. "Vitamin E's Powerful Family Of Antioxidants."

39) Watkins TR, Bierenbaum ML, Giampaolo A. Tocotrienols: Biological and Health Effects. In Antioxidant Status, Diet, Nutrition and Health, Papas AM editor, CRC Press, Boca Raton, 1998;479–96

40) Kooyenga DK, Watkins TR, Geller M, et al. Hypocholesterolemic and antioxidant effects if rice bran oil non-saponifiables in hypercholesterolemic subjects. *Journal of Environmental and Nutritional Interactions* 1999; 3:1–8.

41) Papas, Andreas M. "Vitamin E: a new perspective." AGRO FOOD INDUSTRY HI TECH 12.5 (2001): 23–27. *Douglas Labs Newsletter* 2008

42) Khanna, Savita, et al. "Neuroprotective properties of the natural vitamin E α-tocotrienol." *Stroke* 36.10 (2005): e144-e152.

43) Verlangieri, A. J., and M. J. Bush. "Effects of d-alpha-tocopherol supplementation on experimentally induced primate atherosclerosis." Journal of the *American College of Nutrition* 11.2 (1992): 131–138.

44) Hodis, Howard N., et al. "Serial coronary angiographic evidence that antioxidant vitamin intake reduces progression of coronary artery atherosclerosis." Jama 273.23 (1995): 1849–1854.

45) Stephens, Nigel G., et al. "Randomised controlled trial of vitamin E in patients with coronary disease: Cambridge Heart Antioxidant Study (CHAOS)." *The Lancet* 347.9004 (1996): 781–786.

46) Qureshi, Asaf A., et al. "Novel tocotrienols of rice bran inhibit atherosclerotic lesions in C57BL/6 ApoE-deficient mice." The Journal of nutrition 131.10 (2001): 2606–2618.

47) Black, Tracy M., et al. "Palm tocotrienols protect ApoE+/− mice from diet-induced atheroma formation." *The Journal of nutrition* 130.10 (2000): 2420–2426.

48) Shaish, Aviv, et al. "Dietary β-carotene and α-tocopherol combination does not inhibit atherogenesis in an Apoe–deficient mouse model." *Arteriosclerosis, Thrombosis, and Vascular Biology* 19.6 (1999): 1470–1475.

49) Rimm, Eric B., et al. "Vitamin E consumption and the risk of coronary heart disease in men." *New England Journal of Medicine* 328.20 (1993): 1450–1456.

50) Stampfer, Meir J., et al. "Vitamin E consumption and the risk of coronary disease in women." *New England Journal of Medicine* 328.20 (1993): 1444–1449.

51) Hickey, Steve, and Hilary Roberts. *Ascorbate: The science of vitamin C.* Lulu. com, 2004.

52) Natural Vitamin E Dramatically Reduces Heart Disease by Byron J. Richards, CCN August 17, 2007, NewsWithViews.com

53) Boaz, M., et al. "Secondary prevention with antioxidants of cardiovascular disease in endstage renal disease (SPACE): randomised placebo-controlled trial." *The Lancet* 356.9237 (2000): 1213–1218.

Atherosclerotic Plaque as Infected Biofilm

AT THE COMMERCIAL EXHIBIT AREA at a medical conference in Hollywood, Florida, I had the good fortune to meet Dr. Stephen Fry. We chatted about his latest discoveries in the field of microbiology using the latest techniques, such as the 16s Ribosome technique. Dr. Fry's lab uses this technology to examine atherosclerotic plaque material obtained from surgery. (1–2) Dr. Fry's lab has identified bacterial, fungal, and parasitic DNA in the atherosclerotic plaque samples. (16–18) His findings have been confirmed by other labs. (3)(7–8) Their discovery of atherosclerotic plaque as infected biofilm creates a paradigm shift in our thinking about atherosclerosis.

Stephen Fry Lab: Leaky Gut and LPS

With the recent revelations of Allesio Fasano et al. about the increased permeability of the gut wall called "Leaky Gut," which allows bacterial organisms and undigested food particles into the bloodstream, the next logical thought in this sequence is: *What happens to all these micro-organisms that are leaking into the bloodstream?* (10–13)

Undoubtedly, there is an immune response with release of inflammatory cytokines. In addition, since of these microbial organisms possess amino acid sequences similar to those of our own tissues, this "leakage" may trigger autoimmune disease through the wonders of "molecular mimicry." (19) (20) However, my question is: *"What happens when these micro-organisms set up house? Where do they go, and what do they do?"*

Endothelium as the Innocent Bystander

Of course, blood flowing from the GI tract, "the gut," enters the portal venous system, which goes directly to the liver and spleen. The reticuloendothelial system of the liver and spleen serve as a giant filtering system for all the particles leaking into the bloodstream from our permeable small bowels. This is protective. However, assuming this filtering system has been overwhelmed, allowing a bolus of slimy micro-organisms to gain entry to circulation, where does it go? It goes into the wall of the artery. Setting up house in the arterial wall, the endothelium (the inner lining), or the media (the middle layer) of our blood vessels, is not difficult to imagine. After all, the arterial wall is in direct contact with our evil bolus of micro-organisms. Not only that, the arterial wall is fed by its own blood supply courtesy of capillaries in the vasa vasorum, which may seed microorganisms if present in the circulation.(21) Recent studies reveal angiogenesis, growth of new blood vessels in the vasa vasorum as integral to atherosclerotic pathology.(22) Could this angiogenesis be a tissue response to infection seeded into the wall of the vessel? We await further studies on this.

Injury Leading to Infection

Any injury, scrape, laceration, or break in the dermal barrier, the skin, allows the entry of micro-organisms, which then form an infection, with the usual hallmarks of pus and inflammation. The same can be said for the vascular system. Formation of atherosclerotic plaque tends to occur at sites of injury; at the bifurcations, where shear forces are at their greatest; and at sites of movement like the coronary arteries embedded in the moving surface of the left ventricle. (14) So, the idea of atherosclerotic plaque as infected biofilm certainly fits the pattern of commonly affected sites in the arterial tree.

Plaque as Infected Biofilm: Uffe Ravnskov and Killmer McKully

Uffe Ravnskov and Killmer McKully have been writing about infection in atherosclerotic plaque for years. (5–6) These two doctors amassed evidence that atherosclerotic plaque is an infected biofilm colonized with a diverse flora of bacterial, fungal, and protozoal organisms.

Dr. Ravnskov reminds us of Dr. Hecht's coronary calcium score study. In this study of 930 consecutive asymptomatic patients on no meds and no history of heart disease, Dr. Hecht reported the coronary calcium scores showed no correlation with serum cholesterol levels, providing strong evidence against the cholesterol theory of heart disease. (15)

The End for Statins?

If atherosclerotic plaque is infected biofilm, then this represents a paradigm shift in our thinking about the etiology of atherosclerotic vascular disease and the end of the anti-cholesterol statin drug era. OOPS! The drug industry is not going to be happy about this one.

◆　◆　◆　◆　◆

◆ References for Chapter 12

1) Fry, Stephen Eugene, et al. "Putative biofilm-forming organisms in the human vasculature: expanded case reports and review of the literature." *Phlebological Review* 22.1 (2014): 24–37.

2) Stephen Fry Interview on Biofilms and Protomyxzoa Rheumatica Marc Braman

3) Lanter, Bernard B., Karin Sauer, and David G. Davies. "Bacteria present in carotid arterial plaques are found as biofilm deposits which may contribute to enhanced risk of plaque rupture." *MBio* 5.3 (2014): e01206–14.

4) Schor, Jacob. Alschuler, Lise. "Bacterial Growth in Arteries Implicated in Heart Attacks Stress, biofilms, and cardiovascular disease." August 2014 Vol. 6 Issue 8 *Natural Medicine Journal.*

5) Ravnskov, Uffe, and Kilmer S. McCully. "Biofilms, Lipoprotein Aggregates, Homocysteine, and Arterial Plaque Rupture." *mBio* 5.5 (2014): e01717–14.

6) Ravnskov, U., and K. S. McCully. "Infections may be causal in the pathogenesis of atherosclerosis." *The American journal of the medical sciences* 344.5 (2012): 391.

7) Ott, Stephan J., et al. "Detection of diverse bacterial signatures in atherosclerotic lesions of patients with coronary heart disease." *Circulation* 113.7 (2006): 929–937.

8) Ott, Stephan J., et al. "Fungal rDNA signatures in coronary atherosclerotic plaques." Environmental microbiology 9.12 (2007): 3035-3045.

9) Vojdani, A. "The Role of Periodontal Disease and Other Infections in the Pathogenesis of Atherosclerosis and Systemic Diseases." *Townsend Letter for Doctors and Patients* (2000): 52–57.

10) Fasano, Alessio. "Zonulin, regulation of tight junctions, and autoimmune diseases." *Annals of the New York Academy of Sciences* 1258.1 (2012): 25–33.

11) Fasano, Alessio. "Zonulin and its regulation of intestinal barrier function: the biological door to inflammation, autoimmunity, and cancer." *Physiological reviews* 91.1 (2011): 151–175.

13) Moreno-Navarrete, José María, et al. "Circulating zonulin, a marker of intestinal permeability, is increased in association with obesity-associated insulin resistance." *PloS one* 7.5 (2012): e37160.

14) Asakura, Toshihisa, and Takeshi Karino. "Flow patterns and spatial distribution of atherosclerotic lesions in human coronary arteries." *Circulation research* 66.4 (1990): 1045–1066.

15) Hecht, Harvey S., et al. "Relation of coronary artery calcium identified by electron beam tomography to serum lipoprotein levels and implications for treatment." *American Journal of Cardiology* 87.4 (2001): 406–412.

16) Poonawala, Husain, and David Peaper. "Bacterial Identification using 16S rRNA Gene Sequencing in a University Teaching Hospital." *Open forum infectious diseases*. Vol. 4. No. Suppl 1. Oxford University Press, 2017.

17) Watts, George S., et al. "16S rRNA gene sequencing on a benchtop sequencer: accuracy for identification of clinically important bacteria." *Journal of applied microbiology* 123.6 (2017): 1584–1596.

18) Salipante, Stephen J., et al. "Rapid 16S rRNA next-generation sequencing of polymicrobial clinical samples for diagnosis of complex bacterial infections." *PloS one* 8.5 (2013): e65226.

19) Cusick, Matthew F., Jane E. Libbey, and Robert S. Fujinami. "Molecular mimicry as a mechanism of autoimmune disease." *Clinical reviews in allergy & immunology* 42.1 (2012): 102–111.

20) Doxey, Andrew C., and Brendan J. McConkey. "Prediction of molecular mimicry candidates in human pathogenic bacteria." *Virulence* 4.6 (2013): 453–466.

21) Xu, Junyan, Xiaotong Lu, and Guo-Ping Shi. "Vasa vasorum in atherosclerosis and clinical significance." International journal of molecular sciences 16.5 (2015): 11574-11608.

22) Wu, Wen, et al. "The Role of Angiogenesis in Coronary Artery Disease: A Double-edged Sword: Intraplaque Angiogenesis in Physiopathology and Therapeutic Angiogenesis for Treatment." Current pharmaceutical design 24.4 (2018): 451-464.

CHAPTER

13

Low-Level Endotoxemia-LPS Theory
of Coronary Artery Disease

THE LPS THEORY OF CORONARY artery disease is the idea that "leaky gut" is the direct cause of atherosclerosis by virtue of the LPS, the endotoxin released into the bloodstream that incites an inflammatory reaction in the endothelium. (28–33) LPS is short for Lipopolysaccharide, the outer lipid coat of gram-negative microbial organisms residing in the GI tract. Studies show that a low level of endotoxemia is common in this population, and the level of LPS in the bloodstream correlates with the risk of cardiovascular disease. (33)

Prevent Leaky Gut to Prevent Vascular Disease

Various interventions to prevent leaky gut have been shown to also reduce the progression of atherosclerosis. One such study from April 2016 by Dr. Lin showed that in mice genetically engineered for accelerated atherosclerosis, treatment with a probiotic that restores the mucin barrier and prevents leaky gut also serves to reduce atherosclerosis. The authors state:

The probiotic akermansia muciniphila, attenuates atherosclerotic lesions by ameliorating metabolic endotoxemia-induced inflammation through restoration of the gut barrier. (1)

According to Dr. Brown in a 2015 article, the circulating endotoxin "metabolic endotoxemia" is prevalent in many chronic metabolic diseases, such as obesity, type II diabetes, and atherosclerosis. (4) Increased intestinal permeability, leaky gut, and low-level endotoxemia have also been implicated in Parkinson's Disease, a neurodegenerative condition. (26–27)

LPS Endotoxemia and Atherosclerotic Heart Disease

Dr. Lehr showed that endotoxin-treated rabbits exhibited accelerated atherosclerosis. (5,6). In the human population, the Bruneck study established low-level endotoxemia and systemic inflammation as a strong predictor for atherosclerosis. (33)

Animal Models

The LPS-induced animal model of atherosclerosis has emerged as a popular laboratory technique to test various interventions in mice genetically engineered for atherosclerosis (ApoE mouse). Dr. Cuaz-Pérolin reported in 2008 that weekly LPS injections in mice doubled the atherosclerotic plaque size. Treatment with various anti-inflammatory botanicals (such as Boswellia) cut plaque size in half. (14)

Other Substances Beneficial in the LPS ApoE Mouse Model

These nutritional supplements are all useful for reducing plaque size in the genetically modified mouse model of atherosclerosis (14–22):

- Anthocyanins from sweet potato
- Bee venom
- Bilberry extract
- Fish oil
- Garlic
- Liposomal glutathione
- Stress reduction
- Tocotrienol vitamin E
- Vitamin C.

Now that the cholesterol theory of atherosclerotic heart disease has been shown to be false, we are free to direct attention to the true cause of athero-sclerotic vascular disease: leaky gut with low-level endotoxemia and systemic inflammation. Prevention of atherosclerosis should focus on interventions that block leaky gut and reduce low-level endotoxemia and the associated systemic inflammation.

♦ ♦ ♦ ♦ ♦

♦ References for Chapter 13

1) Li J, Lin S, Vanhoutte PM, Woo CW, Xu A. Akkermansia muciniphila protects against atherosclerosis by preventing metabolic endotoxemia induced inflammation in Apoe-/- mice. *Circulation.* April 2016. pii: Circulation AHA. 115.019645.

2) Bland, Jeffrey. "Intestinal Microbiome, Akkermansia muciniphila, and Medical Nutrition Therapy." Integrative Medicine: A Clinician's Journal 15.5 (2016). Intestinal Microbiome, Akkermansia muciniphila, and Medical Nutrition Therapy.

3) Yamashita, Tomoya, et al. "Gut Microbiota and Coronary Artery Disease." *International Heart Journal* 57.6 (2016): 663–671.

4) Brown, J. Mark, and Stanley L. Hazen. "The Gut Microbial Endocrine Organ: Bacterially-Derived Signals Driving Cardiometabolic Diseases." *Annual review of medicine* 66 (2015): 343.

5) Neves AL, Coelho J, Couto L, et al. Metabolic endotoxemia: a molecular link between obesity and cardiovascular disease. 2013;51:R51–64.

6) Lehr, Hans-Anton, et al. "Immunopathogenesis of atherosclerosis Endotoxin accelerates atherosclerosis in rabbits on hypercholesterolemic diet." *Circulation* 104.8 (2001): 914–920.

7) Rice, James B., et al. "Low-level endotoxin induces potent inflammatory activation of human blood vessels inhibition by statins." Arteriosclerosis, thrombosis, and vascular biology 23.9 (2003): 1576–1582.

8) Stoll, Lynn L., Gerene M. Denning, and Neal L. Weintraub. "Potential role of endotoxin as a proinflammatory mediator of atherosclerosis." Arteriosclerosis, thrombosis, and vascular biology 24.12 (2004): 2227–2236.

9) Manco, Melania, Lorenza Putignani, and Gian Franco Bottazzo. "Gut microbiota, lipopolysaccharides, and innate immunity in the pathogenesis of obesity and cardiovascular risk." *Endocrine reviews* 31.6 (2010): 817–844.

10) Szeto, Cheuk-Chun, et al. "Endotoxemia is related to systemic inflammation and atherosclerosis in peritoneal dialysis patients." *Clinical Journal of the American Society of Nephrology* 3.2 (2008): 431–436.

11) McIntyre, Christopher W., et al. "Circulating endotoxemia: a novel factor in systemic inflammation and cardiovascular disease in chronic kidney disease." *Clinical Journal of the American Society of Nephrology* 6.1 (2011): 133–141.

12) Horseman, Michael, Salim Surani, and John D Bowman. "Endotoxin, Toll-like Receptor-4, and atherosclerotic heart disease." *Current cardiology reviews* 13.2 (2017): 86–93.

13) Kiechl, Stefan, et al. "Toll-like receptor 4 polymorphisms and atherogenesis." *New England Journal of Medicine* 347.3 (2002): 185–192.

14) Cuaz-Pérolin, Clarisse, et al. "Antiinflammatory and antiatherogenic effects of the NF-κB inhibitor acetyl-11-keto-β-boswellic acid in LPS-challenged ApoE−/− mice." *Arteriosclerosis, thrombosis, and vascular biology* 28.2 (2008): 272–277.

15) Gonen, Ayelet, et al. "The antiatherogenic effect of allicin: possible mode of action." *Pathobiology* 72.6 (2005): 325–334.

16) Wang, Hsueh-Hsiao, et al. "Fish oil increases antioxidant enzyme activities in macrophages and reduces atherosclerotic lesions in apoE-knockout mice." *Cardiovascular research* 61.1 (2004): 169–176.

17) Rosenblat, Mira, et al. "Anti-oxidant and anti-atherogenic properties of liposomal glutathione: studies in vitro, and in the atherosclerotic apolipoprotein E-deficient mice." *Atherosclerosis* 195.2 (2007): e61-e68.

18) Miyazaki, Kouji, et al. "Anthocyanins from purple sweet potato Ipomoea batatas cultivar Ayamurasaki suppress the development of atherosclerotic lesions and both enhancements of oxidative stress and soluble vascular cell adhesion molecule-1 in apolipoprotein E-deficient mice." *Journal of agricultural and food chemistry* 56.23 (2008): 11485–11492.

19) Mauray, Aurelie, et al. "Atheroprotective effects of bilberry extracts in apo E-deficient mice." *Journal of agricultural and food chemistry* 57.23 (2009): 11106–11111.

20) Qureshi, Asaf A., et al. "Novel tocotrienols of rice bran inhibit atherosclerotic lesions in C57BL/6 ApoE-deficient mice." *The Journal of nutrition* 131.10 (2001): 2606–2618.

21) Ni, Mei, et al. "Atherosclerotic plaque disruption induced by stress and lipopolysaccharide in apolipoprotein E knockout mice." American Journal of Physiology-Heart and Circulatory Physiology 296.5 (2009): H1598-H1606.

22) Kim, S. J., et al. "The Protective Effect of Apamin on LPS/Fat-Induced Atherosclerotic Mice." Evidence-based complementary and alternative medicine: *eCAM* 2012 (2011): 305454–305454.

23) Chistiakov, Dmitry A., et al. "Role of gut microbiota in the modulation of atherosclerosis-associated immune response." *Frontiers in microbiology* 6 (2015).

24) Ostos, Maria A., et al. "Implication of natural killer t cells in atherosclerosis development during a LPS-induced chronic inflammation." *FEBS letters* 519.1–3 (2002): 23–29.

25) Babaev, Vladimir R., et al. "Combined Vitamin C and Vitamin E Deficiency Worsens Early Atherosclerosis in ApoE-Deficient Mice." *Arteriosclerosis, thrombosis, and vascular biology* 30.9 (2010): 1751.

26) Glaros, Trevor G., et al. "Causes and consequences of low grade endotoxemia and inflammatory diseases." *Front Biosci* (Schol Ed) 5 (2013): 754–765.

27) Houser, Madelyn C., and Malú G. Tansey. "The gut-brain axis: is intestinal inflammation a silent driver of Parkinson's disease pathogenesis?." *Parkinson's Disease* 3.1 (2017): 3.

28) Rogler, Gerhard, and Giuseppe Rosano. "The heart and the gut." *European heart journal* 35.7 (2013): 426–430.

29) Ascher, Stefanie, and Christoph Reinhardt. "The gut microbiota–an emerging risk factor for cardiovascular and cerebrovascular disease." *European journal of immunology* (2017).

30) Pastori, Daniele, et al. "Gut-Derived Serum Lipopolysaccharide is Associated With Enhanced Risk of Major Adverse Cardiovascular Events in Atrial Fibrillation: Effect of Adherence to Mediterranean Diet." *Journal of the American Heart Association* 6.6 (2017): e005784.

31) Ibrahim, Mohamed, et al. "Cardiovascular risk of circulating endotoxin level in prevalent hemodialysis patients." *The Egyptian Heart Journal* (2017).

32) Carnevale, Roberto, et al. "Localization of lipopolysaccharide from Escherichia Coli into human atherosclerotic plaque." *Scientific reports* 8.1 (2018): 3598.

33) Wiedermann CJ, Kiechl S, Dunzendorfer S, et al. Association of endotoxemia with carotid atherosclerosis and cardiovascular disease: prospective results from the Bruneck Study. *J Am Coll Cardiol.* 1999;34(7):1975–81.

NSAIDS, Leaky Gut, and Heart Disease

JIM TAKES NON-STEROIDAL ANTI-INFLAMMATORY DRUGS (NSAIDs)—
ibuprofen, indomethacin, or naproxen—on a regular basis for his arthritis
pain. In addition, Jim's calcium score is very high. Jim had a coronary stent
placed for chest pain about 5 years ago during cardiac catheterization. Jim
wants to know why he should stop the pain pills and switch to a safer and
more effective botanical alternative.

The Vioxx Scandal—A 4.85 Billion Settlement

NSAID drugs have been associated with increased heart attacks for
many years now. (1–9) The 2000 "Vioxx Scandal" was due to the increased
heart-attack rate discovered many years after introduction of a new NSAID
drug called rofecoxib (Vioxx). In November 2007, Merck announced a $4.85
billion settlement, the largest drug settlement in drug history, with 47,000
plaintiffs who had claimed that Vioxx had caused their heart attack. (10)

All NSAIDS Cause Heart Attacks

However, this problem is not restricted to Vioxx. In fact, all NSAID drugs
are associated with increased heart-attack risk, according to a recent publication in the *British Medical Journal*. (2) What is the mechanism by which
NSAIDS causes heart attacks? None of the medical publications take the next
step of explaining this. (2–9) In my opinion, the obvious explanation is that
NSAIDs cause leaky gut with low-level endotoxemia.

NSAIDS Cause Leaky Gut

There is overwhelming evidence that NSAIDS cause of leaky gut. (1) Animal studies show NSAID-induced damage to the small bowel intestinal brush border, with increased intestinal permeability and "leaky gut" in virtually all animals treated with NSAIDS. (17–19)

Leaky Gut Causes Heart Disease

The previous chapter on the low-level endotoxemia-LPS theory of heart disease explains the mechanism by which leaky gut causes low-level endotoxemia, a known risk factor for coronary artery disease and increased risk for heart attacks. Low-level endotoxemia is the fancy medical name for leakage of gut bacteria into the bloodstream. This has been directly linked to causing atherosclerotic plaque, a form of infected biofilm discussed in my previous article on this topic.

Dr. Michelle Bally writes in a 2017 article in *BMJ*:

All NSAIDs, including naproxen, were found to be associated with an increased risk of acute myocardial infarction. (2)

NSAIDS Are Mitochondrial Toxins

Another adverse effect of NSAIDS is that they are mitochondrial toxins that target sensitive myocardial muscle cells, causing 20% of hospital admissions for congestive heart failure. (15–16) NSAIDS have been shown to uncouple oxidative phosphorylation in mitochondria. Thus, small-bowel damage by NSAID drugs is explained as a "topical effect" of the drug-producing mitochondrial damage in the cells that line the gut, the enterocytes. (17–19)

Athletes' Sudden Death from Coronary Artery Disease

"Cardiac arrest is the leading cause of death in young athletes, but the incidence of it is unclear." (24-26) Strenuous exercise itself can cause leaky gut with endotoxemia, as reported in a number of studies of athletes. (21) In

addition, serious liver enzyme elevation can occur after strenuous exercise, probably from the endotoxins released from the gut that travel to the liver. (22) This makes athletes susceptible to coronary artery disease. The risk is increased if the athlete takes NSAIDS for musculoskeletal injuries after exercise. (23)

Summary

The obvious mechanism by which NSAID drugs cause coronary artery disease and increased heart-attack risk is leaky gut. This allows leakage of LPS and gram-negative bacteria into the bloodstream, a form of low-level endotoxemia directly linked to atherosclerotic disease. Avoiding NSAID drugs is essential for healing the gut and preventing coronary artery disease.

♦ ♦ ♦ ♦ ♦

♦ References for Chapter 14

1) NSAIDS, Small Bowel and Leaky Gut by Jeffrey Dach MD

2) Bally, Michèle, et al. "Risk of acute myocardial infarction with NSaids in real world use: Bayesian meta-analysis of individual patient data." *BMJ* 357 (2017): j1909.

3) Johnsen, Søren P., et al. "Risk of hospitalization for myocardial infarction among users of rofecoxib, celecoxib, and other NSAIDs: a population-based case-control study." *Archives of internal medicine* 165.9 (2005): 978–984.

4) Olsen, Anne-Marie Schjerning, et al. "Long-term cardiovascular risk of NSAID use according to time passed after first-time myocardial infarction: a nationwide cohort study." *Circulation* (2012): CIRCULATIONAHA-112.

5) Leaky Gut Syndrome Isn't Only Scary, But Extremely Dangerous to Your Health – This is More Than a Poop Issue! by Jordan Reasoner

6) Kohli, Payal, et al. "NSAID use and association with cardiovascular outcomes in outpatients with stable atherothrombotic disease." *The American journal of medicine* 127.1 (2014): 53–60.

7) "Common painkillers may raise risk of heart attack by 100% – study. Risk of myocardial infarction is greatest in first month of taking NSAIDs such as ibuprofen if dose is high, say researchers." By Haroon Siddique *The Guardian*, May 2017

8) "Calls for ibuprofen sale restrictions after study finds cardiac arrest risk. Over-the-counter drug linked to 31% increased cardiac arrest risk, with the figure rising to 50% for diclofenac, says research." By Matthew Weaver, *The Guardian*, Mar 2017

9) "FDA strengthens warning that NSAIDs increase heart attack and stroke risk," July 13, 2015 Gregory Curfman, MD, Editor in Chief, Harvard Health Publications

10) Special Series. "Vioxx: The Downfall of a Drug" NPR, November 9, 2007.

11) NSAIDs Causing Heart Attacks? Guide to the Perplexed. By Dov Michaeli, MD, PhD -June 30, 2012

12) Opioid Wars: Opioids vs. NSAIDs Cathryn Jakobson Ramin December 08, 2015

13) NSAIDs May Increase Heart Attack Risk Gabe Mirkin MD

14) NSAIDs and Cardiovascular Risk Explained, According to Studies from the Perelman School of Medicine May 02, 2012 Philadelphia

15) Ghosh, Rajeshwary, Azra Alajbegovic, and Aldrin V. Gomes. "NSAIDs and cardiovascular diseases: role of reactive oxygen species." *Oxidative medicine and cellular longevity* 2015 (2015).

16) Page, John, and David Henry. "Consumption of NSAIDs and the development of congestive heart failure in elderly patients: an underrecognized public health problem." *Archives of internal medicine* 160.6 (2000): 777–784.

17) Somasundaram, S., et al. "Mitochondrial damage: a possible mechanism of the" topical" phase of NSAID induced injury to the rat intestine." *Gut* 41.3 (1997): 344.

18) Somasundaram, S., et al. "Uncoupling of intestinal mitochondrial oxidative phosphorylation and inhibition of cyclooxygenase are required for the development of NSAID-enteropathy in the rat." *Alimentary Pharmacology and Therapeutics* 14.5 (2000): 639.

19) Matsui, Hirofumi, et al. "The pathophysiology of non-steroidal anti-inflammatory drug (NSAID)-induced mucosal injuries in stomach and small intestine." *Journal of Clinical Biochemistry and Nutrition* 48.2 (2011): 107.

20) Ashton, Tony, et al. "Exercise-induced endotoxemia: the effect of ascorbic acid supplementation." *Free Radical Biology and Medicine* 35.3 (2003): 284–291.

21) Bosenberg, A. T., et al. "Strenuous exercise causes systemic endotoxemia." Journal of Applied Physiology 65.1 (1988): 106-108.

22) Pettersson, Jonas, et al. "Muscular exercise can cause highly pathological liver function tests in healthy men." British journal of clinical pharmacology 65.2 (2008): 253-259.

23) Van Wijck, Kim, et al. "Aggravation of exercise-induced intestinal injury by Ibuprofen in athletes." Medicine & Science in Sports & Exercise 44.12 (2012): 2257-2262.

24) Sweeting, Joanna, and Christopher Semsarian. "Sudden cardiac death in athletes: still much to learn." Cardiology clinics 34.4 (2016): 531-541.

25) Wasfy, Meagan M., Adolph M. Hutter, and Rory B. Weiner. "Sudden cardiac death in athletes." Methodist DeBakey cardiovascular journal 12.2 (2016): 76.

26) Semsarian, Christopher, Joanna Sweeting, and Michael J. Ackerman. "Sudden cardiac death in athletes." Br J Sports Med 49.15 (2015): 1017-1023.

CHAPTER	Reverse Heart Disease with the
15	Coronary Calcium Score

FOR MANY YEARS, THE AMERICAN Heart Association denied that coronary calcium scoring is a valid marker for heart disease risk. They have finally admitted the coronary calcium score reliably predicts heart-attack risk. (1) UCLA cardiologist Dr. Matt Budoff, a long-time champion of the coronary calcium scan, and author of an AHA paper, says:

The total amount of coronary calcium predicts coronary disease events beyond standard risk factors. (1)

In a 2008 *New England Journal* article, Dr. Robert Detrano states:

The coronary calcium score is a strong predictor of incident coronary heart disease and provides predictive information beyond that provided by standard risk factors. (31)

The Coronary Calcium Score is a precise quantitative tool for measuring and tracking heart disease risk and is more valuable and accurate than other traditional markers, such as total cholesterol, which is practically worthless as a predictor of heart disease risk.

What Is Coronary Artery Disease? It's Plaque Formation.

In youth, there is minimal plaque formation in our arteries. However, with the passage of time, arterial plaque grows larger. About 20% of this plaque volume contains calcium, which is measurable on a CAT scan, providing a marker for the total plaque burden. Calcium score, and by inference, plaque volume, typically increases 30–35% per year in untreated patients.

As we age, the enlarging plaque may eventually obstruct blood flow caus-ing myocardial ischemia, or even worse, occlusion with heart attack. Another common scenario is plaque rupture, which exposes the inflammatory debris of the plaque to the circulating blood. This quickly results in clot formation, also called thrombosis, resulting in a heart attack and possibly sudden death. The calcified portion of the plaque is consistently 20% of the total plaque volume, allowing use of the calcium score as an accurate marker for total plaque volume.

Annual Calcium Score Progression

An even more useful tool is the annual calcium score progression calcu-lated from two annual scans. Annual calcium score progression of less than 15% per year is associated with benign prognosis. Progression above 15% per year is associated with poor prognosis and high risk for future heart attack. (12)

Arterial Calcification – Why Does It Happen?

Calcification in the soft tissues (connective tissue, ligaments, muscles, arteries) is found in many disease states and is commonly identified on pathology slides of tissues.

The most common cause of soft-tissue calcification is bacterial, fungal, or parasitic infection. Examples include:

Egg-shell calcification in the pericardium results from tuberculous pericarditis.

Punctate calcifications in the lungs called calcified granulomas may result from previous pulmonary fungal disease such as histoplasmosis and coccidiomycosis (Valley Fever).

The parasite cysticercosis produces punctate calcifications in the brain and muscles with a characteristic appearance on a CAT scan.

Hepatic calcifications may be caused by tuberculosis, histoplasmosis, coccidioidomycosis, brucellosis, echinococcal cyst schistosomiasis, cysticercosis, filariasis, paragonimiasis, guinea worm, and chronic amebic and pyogenic abscess. (63)

Wherever inflammation occurs, the body invokes a process of calcification as part of the healing process. Arterial calcification is literally bone formation in the wall of the artery triggered by an inflammatory process or infection. Pathology studies have shown that coronary artery calcium forms in areas of healed plaque ruptures. (21) Calcification and plaque formation increases with age, with the calcium score typically increasing 30–35% per year in untreated patients. There is an increasing heart-attack rate with higher coronary calcium scores.

Calcium Score is Highly Predictive of Heart-Attack Risk

What is a heart attack? A heart attack is the death of heart muscle cells caused by oxygen deprivation from lack of blood flow. As previously mentioned, this is caused by blocking of the feeding artery, thought to be associated with enlarging plaque formation that blocks the lumen, or perhaps plaque rupture that causes clot formation that then blocks the lumen. If a small area of heart muscle is involved, the heart attack may be silent, with no symptoms. If a larger area is involved, there may be severe chest pain radiating to the left arm or jaw, or other symptoms such as shortness of breath. If the conduction system is involved, there may be an irregular heart rhythm called ventricular tachycardia, which can cause sudden death.

A lesser form of disease is called "angina pectoris," which is chest pain without a full-blown heart attack. Angina pectoris is treated with medicines such as nitroglycerine to dilate the arteries.

Common Sites of Plaque Formation: Bifurcations and Sites of Mechanical Stress

Ask any interventional radiologist or invasive cardiologist where they most commonly find the arterial plaque formation and arterial obstructions. (13) They will find the arterial lesions at the same places. These places are the carotid bifurcation, the distal aorta at the bifurcation, the femoral bifurcation, the exit from the adductor canal. And of course, the proximal coronary arteries, and bifurcations of the coronary arteries.

These Y-type bifurcations have maximal turbulence and place the greatest mechanical stress on the vessel wall. Remember, the blood is flowing under pressure, driven by pulsation, and this mechanical pressure and turbulence, over time, causes little stress cracks in the vessel. The cracks appear at these sites of stress. The coronary arteries are a special case, because the extra motion of the cardiac muscle itself moves and stretches the coronary arteries with every cardiac contraction.

The coronary arteries near the aorta are relatively stationary, while lower down over the surface of the heart, the coronary arteries rest on the surface of the heart, moving vigorously with each cardiac contraction. Atherosclerotic plaque typically forms at these locations, where the arterial wall is subject to mechanical stress. (13)

William Davis MD, Advocate of the Coronary Calcium Score

William Davis, MD, author or the *New York Times* bestseller *Wheat Belly* and *Undoctored* is a Wisconsin cardiologist who has written for many years about using the calcium score to reverse heart disease. Dr. Davis recommends screening CAT heart scans in males over 40 and females over 50. He would start at younger ages if high-risk features are present, such as strong family history of early heart disease, cigarette smoking, diabetes mellitus, or severe lipid or lipoprotein genetic disorders. (2–3) The coronary calcium score test is currently covered by Medicare and many health insurances. (32) Credit and thanks is given to William Davis MD at the Track Your Plaque website and to Wheat Belly Blog for much of the information in this chapter. I have taken the liberty to add and modify a few things.

What Does Calcium Look Like?

Calcium in the coronary arteries is easily seen as "white" on the CAT scan and can be measured by the computer to yield a calcium score, which is a quantification of the total calcification.

Review of Benefits of Coronary Calcium Scoring

Calcium scoring may be superior to angiography as a means to track plaque.

Calcium scoring gives a precise number that correlates with the amount of plaque volume. Although only the hard plaque, or calcium, in the artery is actually measured, this is useful because it consistently occupies 20% of plaque volume (total hard and soft plaque).

The new 64-slice CAT scanners provide reliable calcium scoring same as multi-slice and EBT(Electron Beam CAT).

Annual calcium score is useful for calculating progression of calcium score. Annual progression of greater than 15% is associated with poor prognosis, and an annual progression of less than 15% is associated with good prognosis.

Dr. William Davis's Track Your Plaque Program

Quantify plaque with coronary calcium score with CAT scan (or with electron beam CT).

Obtain your CAT scan serially, every 12 months, to assess your response to treatment and lifestyle modification (track your plaque).

Use laboratory testing to assess risk. The lipoprotein panel provides the cholesterol panel, LDL particle size, and number, lipoprotein (a), CRP, and homocysteine level. Repeat every 6 months. (7–8) Note: As mentioned in a previous chapter, LDL cholesterol subfractions are useful in diagnosis of metabolic syndrome; however, LDL subfractions are not reliable predictors of heart-attack risk, and these have been replaced by the serial calcium score.

The main goal of treatment is to reduce the annual progression of the coronary artery calcium score, and by inference, reduce plaque volume and cardiovascular mortality.

How to Measure Success in Halting or Reversing Heart Disease Plaque

Calcium score typically increases at an astonishing rate of 30–35% per year without treatment. Therefore, Dr. Davis considers treatment success to be reduction in this rate from a 30% to perhaps only a 5–10% increase in calcium score per year. Absolute reduction in calcium score on annual follow-up is difficult to achieve. A more achievable and realistic goal is to reduce annual progression to below 15%, which has been found to be associated with a good prognosis in the 2004 Paolo Raggi study. (12)

Cholesterol and Statin Drugs for Calcium Score?

Dr. Hecht and numerous others have shown no correlation between cholesterol level and calcium score. This lack of correlation proves that elevated cholesterol does not cause arterial calcification. Manipulation of cholesterol levels with statin drugs, as mentioned in other chapters, has no beneficial impact on calcium score and is no longer recommended. The adverse side effects of statin drugs may therefore be avoided.

Risk Factors for Coronary Artery Disease and Calcium Score

LDL cholesterol particle size and number. Total cholesterol and LDL Cholesterol do not correlate with coronary calcium score. However, improvement in the LDL cholesterol particle size and number parallel improvement in metabolic syndrome.

Diabetes, or metabolic syndrome. Diabetes, or metabolic syndrome with elevated blood sugar, insulin resistance, elevated CRP, and obesity, represent a profoundly increased risk for accelerated coronary artery disease and rapid annual progression of calcium score (above 30%). The lipoprotein panel may show typical features of metabolic syndrome: elevated small-particle LDL, low HDL, elevated triglycerides, elevated CRP, etc. Achieving normal blood sugar (≤100 mg/dl) with diet and lifestyle modification is important. Diabetes is a high-risk factor for heart disease. Metformin serves as first-line drug treatment for blood-sugar control.

Elevated homocysteine. Elevated homocysteine is treated with B6, B12, and methyl folate.

Elevated lipoprotein(a.) Elevated lipoprotein(a) is a risk factor for accelerated coronary artery disease and should be addressed.

Hypertension. Hypertension is a treatable risk factor. Achieving normal blood pressure (<130/80) is an important part of any program to prevent progression of the calcium score. Even a small elevation of blood pressure in diseased arteries can cause increased mortality.

C-reactive protein. Reduce to normal, under 1 mg/l.

Diet and Lifestyle Modification to Reduce Calcium Score

Not long ago, a 57-year-old man who works on a loading dock came to seem me with a calcium score of 1212. Seven months later, his score had increased to 1650, an 18% increase in less than a year. I started him on the protocol described in this section, and a year later his calcium score was 1543. This patient went from an 18% increase to a decrease of 5%. According to the 2004 Paolo Raggi study, despite having a high starting score, he would be protected from heart attack.

Here is the protocol.

Vitamin K2

The MK4 and MK7 versions of vitamin K2 are the cornerstone of the program to reduce calcium score. See the chapter on vitamin K for more information.

Aged Garlic

Surprisingly, aged garlic is quite beneficial for calcium score and prevents progression effectively. See the chapter on aged garlic for calcium score for more information.

Omega 3 Fish Oil

Fish oil (Omega 3 oils) 3600–4000 mg per day (providing 1200 mg omega-3 fatty acids). (molecular distilled pharmaceutical grade). (36)

Vitamin D3

Vitamin D3 levels should be restored to above 60–70 ng/ml (dosage, Vitamin D3, 5–6,000 u/day based on blood testing). Vitamin K2 (MK-7 and MK-4) is also used along with Vitamin D3. Low vitamin D is associated with increasing arterial calcification and increased heart disease risk. (26) (63–74) Consumption of calcium tablets by women is no longer recommended, as this may increase arterial calcification and heart-attack risk. (5)

Low Glycemic Diet: Eliminate Grains and Sugars

The diet that addresses metabolic syndrome is one that eliminates all grains and sugars, as advocated by Dr. William Davis in his books, *Wheat Belly* and *Undoctored*. As features of metabolic syndrome improve with the new diet, there will be a simultaneous decrease in triglycerides and small-particle LDL, markers for metabolic syndrome. Loss of visceral fat, decreased CRP, and decreased blood pressure are all benefits of new diet.

Avoid sugars and fructose corn syrup, and eliminate wheat products like shredded wheat cereal, Raisin Bran, and whole-wheat bagels. Increase protein intake.

Address Leaky Gut: Testing and Treatment

Leaky gut is commonly found in metabolic syndrome, obesity, and diabetes, and has been implicated in coronary artery disease. Testing for LPS antibodies, antigliadin antibodies and food sensitivities can help demonstrate leaky gut. Treatment of "Leaky Gut" involves a gluten-free organic diet, probiotics, prebiotics, digestive enzymes, berberine, glutamine, zinc, colostrum, etc. (11) Avoid alcohol, NSAID pain pills, and PPI antacids, as these may worsen leaky gut syndrome. (75–83)

Healthy Fats

Consume foods such as raw almonds, walnuts, pecans; cold-pressed olive oil, and avocado oil. Avoid trans-fats, avoid margarines and processed cooking oils etc. Use instead heathy cold-pressed vegetable oils.

Increase Fiber

Ground flaxseed (2 tbsp/day)-Extra fiber aids in detoxifying liver and the entire body by interrupting the enterohepatic circulation.

Vitamin C

Fully buffered vitamin C, 1000–3000 mg/day, is the vitamin for strong collagen formation and strengthens the arterial wall. See chapter 10 on the Linus Pauling protocol, which includes vitamin C and the amino acids proline and lysine, which act as receptors for Lp(a). By consuming additional lysine and proline, the receptor sites on the Lp(a) and other lipoproteins are covered up and made less sticky, resulting in less deposition in the artery wall. The vitamin C is important not only for strong collagen formation, a major component of the arterial wall, but also for all other structural elements of the body. (37)(52-57)

Lifestyle Modification

Exercise and weight loss improve metabolic syndrome and insulin sensitivity, reduce inflammatory markers, and reduce blood pressure. The improvement in lipoprotein profile correlates with improvement in metabolic syndrome. Dietary measures that heal the gut and prevent leaky gut reduce atherosclerotic risk. (86–93)

Magnesium

Magnesium supplementation is inexpensive and safe. Magnesium deficiency due to dietary deficiency or thiazide diuretics for hypertension is common and is associated with increased heart-disease risk. Magnesium reduces blood pressure, relaxes smooth muscle in the arteries, and is needed for normal endothelial function. (41)(42)(43)

L-Arginine

L-arginine is converted to nitric oxide, an important substance for arterial health. Research by Robert Furchgott and others showed that nitric oxide (NO) relaxes arterial smooth muscle, dilating coronary arteries up to 50%. (35) However, NO is gone after a few seconds, so it must be replenished at a constant rate to keep the arteries relaxed and open. Lack of NO is associated with constricted arteries, damage to the arterial lining, and accelerated plaque growth. L-arginine shrinks coronary plaque, corrects "endothelial dysfunction," improves insulin sensitivity, is anti-inflammatory, and shrinks plaque. Dosage: l-arginine 6000 mg twice a day, best taken on an empty stomach.

Tocotrienol Vitamin E

See the chapter on vitamin E for more information on this.

Systemic Enzymes

Serrapeptidase, nattokinase and lumbrokinase are oral-systemic enzyme supplements that may play a role in reducing or slowing progression of the calcium score. They act as fibrinolytic and thrombolytic agents which dissolve blood clots and open closed vessels. Lumbrokinase, a protein from earthworms, is considered the more potent of the three. In 2009, Dr Kasim published his study in 10 patients with stable angina treated for 30 days with lumbrokinase.(62) Six of the ten patients reported reduction in angina symptoms as well as objective evidence of resolution of stress induced myocardial ischemia using perfusion scan with sestamibi. I was very impressed with this, a fertile area for future study.

Reverse Cholesterol Transport and Essential Phospholipid – Phosphatidyl Choline (PC) (38)(39)

James C. Roberts, MD FACC, a cardiologist in Ohio, lectures extensively on his clinical success with phosphatidylcholine (IV or in Liposomal oral form with EDTA). A DVD of his lectures that describes his considerable clinical success with oral EDTA and phosphatidylcholine is available. His web page contains his DVD lecture material, complete with clinical case histories. (61)

Essential phospholipid is available under the trade name Phoschol, which increases lecithin-cholesterol acyl transferase activity (LCAT). (40)(44) Activating LCAT is beneficial because LCAT is the crucial substance that transports cholesterol from the arterial plaque back to the liver for metabolic breakdown into bile. This process reverses atherosclerotic plaque formation. Dosage: 3 softgels of Phoschol a day, each containing 900 mg PC. (38)(39)

Optimizing Thyroid Function

Optimizing thyroid function is highly important for reducing calcium score and atherosclerotic risk. Broda Barnes, MD, showed that low thyroid function markedly increases the risk for coronary artery disease. This conclusion was based on autopsy data from Graz Austria and detailed in his two books, *Hypothyroidism: The Unsuspected Illness*, and *Solved: The Riddle of Heart Attacks.* (59)

A low-thyroid condition is associated with increased susceptibility to infection. If atherosclerotic plaque is infected biofilm seeded by microorganisms from the gut, then optimal thyroid function would defend against such an infectious insult. (94)

Reducing Lipoprotein (a)(2)(3)

Lp(a) is a genetic variant lipoprotein associated with a high risk of heart disease, and therefore identifying and reducing Lp(a) is essential. The problem is that the conventional Lipid panels done in your doctor's office do not include Lp(a). Only the more sophisticated lipoprotein panels include the test for Lp(a).

Treating Lp(a) with Niacin

Use a slow release, over-the-counter (OTC) niacin product such as Nias-pan (Kos Pharmaceuticals), or Slo-Niacin (Upsher-Smith). Both are better tolerated than plain OTC niacin, which may cause hot flushes. Reduce hot flushes by drinking a full glass of water with each niacin gelcap; some find that adding an aspirin tablet to the routine helps to reduce flushing.

Lp(a) and Bio-identical Hormones

Bio-Identical hormones are beneficial for reducing heart disease. In menopausal females, estrogen preparations such as Bi-Est are used. Estrogens have been shown to reduce coronary artery calcium score. (46) In males over 50, bio-identical testosterone cream may lower Lp(a) by as much as 25%. Medical studies show that optimizing testosterone levels in aging males can reduce risk of coronary artery disease by 60%. (47–48) DHEA can promote weight loss and improve insulin sensitivity. (45)

Lp(a) and L-Carnitine

The supplement L-carnitine can be a useful adjunct; 2000–4000 mg per day (1000 mg twice a day) can reduce Lp(a) 7–8%, and occasionally will reduce it up to 20%.

What about Statin Cholesterol-Lowering Drugs?

Dr. William Davis admits that the total cholesterol and the LDL cho-lesterol numbers are of little value in predicting heart-disease risk. And he says that the statin drug side effects, i.e. muscle pain and weakness, are more common in actual practice than the drug advertising suggests, making statin drugs difficult to take for the long term.

♦ ♦ ♦ ♦ ♦

♦ References for Chapter 15

1) Budoff, Matthew J., et al. "Assessment of coronary artery disease by cardiac computed tomography: a scientific statement from the American Heart Association Committee on Cardiovascular Imaging and Intervention, Council on Cardiovascular Radiology and Intervention, and Committee on Cardiac Imaging, Council on Clinical Cardiology." Circulation 114.16 (2006): 1761–1791.

2) William R. Davis, MD, FACC, is author of Track Your Plaque, Wheat Belly, and Undoctored: Why Health Care Has Failed You and How You Can Become Smarter Than Your Doctor

3) http://www.wheatbellyblog.com/2017/11/reduce-heart-scan-score/ William Davis, MD on how to reduce your calcium score.

4) Marcovina, Santica M., et al. "Fish intake, independent of apo (a) size, accounts for lower plasma lipoprotein (a) levels in Bantu fishermen of Tanzania: The Lugalawa Study." Arteriosclerosis, thrombosis, and vascular biology 19.5 (1999): 1250–1256.

5) Bolland, Mark J., et al. "Vascular events in healthy older women receiving calcium supplementation: randomised controlled trial." Bmj 336.7638 (2008): 262–266.

6) Slo Niacin Upsher Smith

7) LipoScience NMR Lipiprotein Analysis

9) Greenland, Philip, et al. "ACCF/AHA 2007 clinical expert consensus document on coronary artery calcium scoring by computed tomography in global cardiovascular risk assessment and in evaluation of patients with chest pain: a report of the American College of Cardiology Foundation Clinical Expert Consensus Task Force (ACCF/AHA Writing Committee to Update the 2000 Expert Consensus Document on Electron Beam Computed Tomography) developed in collaboration with the Society of Atherosclerosis Imaging and Prevention and the Society of. . . ." Journal of the American College of Cardiology 49.3 (2007): 378–402.

10) Pletcher, Mark J., et al. "Using the coronary artery calcium score to predict coronary heart disease events: a systematic review and meta-analysis." Archives of Internal Medicine 164.12 (2004): 1285–1292.

11) Resnick C. Nutritional protocol for the treatment of intestinal permeability defects and related conditions. NMJ, 2010;2(3), 14–23.

12) Raggi, Paolo, Tracy Q. Callister, and Leslee J. Shaw. "Progression of coronary artery calcium and risk of first myocardial infarction in patients receiving cholesterol-lowering therapy." Arteriosclerosis, thrombosis, and vascular biology 24.7 (2004): 1272–1277.

13) Asakura, Toshihisa, and Takeshi Karino. "Flow patterns and spatial distribution of atherosclerotic lesions in human coronary arteries." Circulation research 66.4 (1990): 1045–1066.

14) Jorgens, Joseph, et al. "The significance of coronary calcification." American Journal of Roentgenology 95.3 (1965): 667–672.

15) Kataoka, Masako, et al. "How predictive is breast arterial calcification of cardiovascular disease and risk factors when found at screening mammography?." American journal of roentgenology 187.1 (2006): 73–80.

16) Wexler, Lewis, et al. "Coronary artery calcification: pathophysiology, epidemiology, imaging methods, and clinical implications: a statement for health professionals from the American Heart Association." Circulation 94.5 (1996): 1175–1192.

17) Sangiorgi, Giuseppe, et al. "Arterial calcification and not lumen stenosis is highly correlated with atherosclerotic plaque burden in humans: a histologic study of 723 coronary artery segments using nondecalcifying methodology." Journal of the American College of Cardiology 31.1 (1998): 126–133.

18) Detrano, Robert, et al. "Prognostic value of coronary calcification and angiographic stenoses in patients undergoing coronary angiography." Journal of the American College of Cardiology 27.2 (1996): 285–290.

19) LaMonte, Michael J., et al. "Coronary artery calcium score and coronary heart disease events in a large cohort of asymptomatic men and women." American journal of epidemiology 162.5 (2005): 421–429.

20) Budoff, Matthew J., et al. "Long-term prognosis associated with coronary calcification: observations from a registry of 25,253 patients." Journal of the American College of Cardiology 49.18 (2007): 1860–1870.

21) Divakaran, S., et al. "Use of cardiac CT and calcium scoring for detecting coronary plaque: implications on prognosis and patient management." The British journal of radiology 88.1046 (2015): 20140594.

22) Redberg, Rita F. "Response to Letter Regarding Article,"Coronary Artery Calcium: Should We Rely on This Surrogate Marker?."" Circulation 114.5 (2006): e83-e83.

23) McCarthy, J. H., and F. J. Palmer. "Incidence and significance of coronary artery calcification." British heart journal 36.5 (1974): 499.

24) Keelan, Paul C., et al. "Long-term prognostic value of coronary calcification detected by electron-beam computed tomography in patients undergoing coronary angiography." Circulation 104.4 (2001): 412–417.

25) Prat-Gonzalez, Susanna, Javier Sanz, and Mario J. Garcia. "Cardiac CT: indications and limitations." Journal of nuclear medicine technology 36.1 (2008): 18–24.

26) Watson, Karol E., et al. "Active serum vitamin D levels are inversely correlated with coronary calcification." Circulation 96.6 (1997): 1755–1760.

27) Loecker, Thomas H., et al. "Fluoroscopic coronary artery calcification and associated coronary disease in asymptomatic young men." Journal of the American College of Cardiology 19.6 (1992): 1167–1172.

28) Colhoun, Helen M., et al. "Lipoprotein subclasses and particle sizes and their relationship with coronary artery calcification in men and women with and without type 1 diabetes." Diabetes 51.6 (2002): 1949–1956.

29) Sacks, Frank M., and Hannia Campos. "Low-density lipoprotein size and cardiovascular disease: a reappraisal." The Journal of Clinical Endocrinology & Metabolism 88.10 (2003): 4525–4532.

30) deleted

31) Detrano, Robert, et al. "Coronary calcium as a predictor of coronary events in four racial or ethnic groups." New England Journal of Medicine 358.13 (2008): 1336–1345.

32) Medicare to Keep Paying for Heart Scans. by Reed Abelson, March 12, 2008 New York Times

33) Cholesterol Lowering Statin Drugs for Women Just Say No to Statin Drugs by Jeffrey Dach MD

34) Lipitor and The Dracula of Modern Technology by Jeffrey Dach MD

35) Nobel Prize in Physiology or Medicine for 1998 jointly to Robert F. Furchgott, Louis J. Ignarro and Ferid Murad for their discoveries concerning "nitric oxide as a signaling molecule in the cardiovascular system." L-Arginine is converted to Nitric Oxide. Press Release NOBELFÖRSAMLINGEN Karolinska Institutet October 12, 1998

36) EPA/DHA ultra-pure

37) Linus Pauling Protocol Short Version for prevention, reversal of heart disease

38) Essential Phospholipid, PhosChol® is 100 percent pure polyenylphosphatidylcholine (PPC), with up to 52% DLPC.

39) Source for PPC, 3 PhosChol capsules delivers 2700mgs of purified PPC.

40) Sparks, Daniel L., et al. "Effect of the cholesterol content of reconstituted LpA-I on lecithin: cholesterol acyltransferase activity." Journal of Biological Chemistry 270.10 (1995): 5151–5157.

41) Berkelhammer, C., and R. A. Bear. "A clinical approach to common electrolyte problems: 4. Hypomagnesemia." Canadian Medical Association Journal 132.4 (1985): 360.

42) Bilbey, D. L., and Victor M. Prabhakaran. "Muscle cramps and magnesium deficiency." Canadian Family Physician 42 (1996): 1348.

43) Elin, Ronald J. "Magnesium metabolism in health and disease." Disease-a-month 34.4 (1988): 166–218.

44) Dobiasova, M., J. Stribrna, and K. Matousovic. "Effect of polyenoic phospholipid therapy on lecithin cholesterol acyltransferase activity in the human serum." Physiologia Bohemoslovaca 37.2 (1988): 165–172.

45) Villareal, Dennis T., and John O. Holloszy. "Effect of DHEA on abdominal fat and insulin action in elderly women and men: a randomized controlled trial." Jama 292.18 (2004): 2243–2248.

46) Manson, JoAnn E., et al. "Estrogen therapy and coronary-artery calcification." New England Journal of Medicine 356.25 (2007): 2591–2602.

47) Bhasin, Shalender, and Karen Herbst. "Testosterone and atherosclerosis progression in men." (2003): 1929–1931.

48) Hak, A. Elisabeth, et al. "Low levels of endogenous androgens increase the risk of atherosclerosis in elderly men: the Rotterdam study." The Journal of Clinical Endocrinology & Metabolism 87.8 (2002): 3632–3639.

49) Levy, Thomas E. Stop America's# 1 Killer!: Reversible Vitamin Deficiency Found to be Origin of All Coronary Heart Disease. LivOn Books, 2006.

50) Levy, Thomas E. Curing the incurable: vitamin C, infectious diseases, and toxins. Livon Books, 2002.

51) Hickey, Steve, and Hilary Roberts. Ascorbate: The science of vitamin C. Lulu. com, 2004.

52) http://www.paulingtherapy.com/ Linus Pauling Protocol for prevention and reversal of heart disease

53) Patent: Prevention and Treatment of Occlusive Cardiovascular Disease with Ascorbate and Substances That Inhibit the Binding if Lipoprotein (a). Inventors: Matthias W. Rath, 7141 Kirchberg/Murr Linus C. Pauling, Big Sur, CA 93920 Patent Application Number: 557,516.

54) Rath, Matthias, and Linus Pauling. "A unified theory of human cardiovascular disease leading the way to the abolition of this disease as a cause for human mortality." Journal of Orthomolecular Medicine 7.1 (1992): 5–15.

55) Rath, Matthias, and Linus Pauling. "Hypothesis: lipoprotein (a) is a surrogate for ascorbate." Proceedings of the National Academy of Sciences 87.16 (1990): 6204–6207.

56) Rath, Matthias, and Linus Pauling. "Immunological evidence for the accumulation of lipoprotein (a) in the atherosclerotic lesion of the hypoascorbemic guinea pig." Proceedings of the National Academy of Sciences 87.23 (1990): 9388–9390.

57) Pauling L, Rath M. Solution to the puzzle of human cardiovascular disease: its primary cause is ascorbate deficiency leading to the deposition of lipoprotein(a) and fibrinogen/fibrin in the vascular wall. J Orthomol Med. 1992;6:125–133.

58) Vitamin C and Stroke Prevention by Jeffrey Dach MD

59) Hypothyroidism the Unsuspected Illness, by Broda Barnes MD, review by Jeffrey Dach MD

60) Vitamin D Deficiency by Jeffrey Dach MD

61) James C. Roberts MD FACC. clinical success with Phosphatidylcholine(IV or in Liposomal Oral Format with EDTA): Reverse Cholesterol Transport and Metal Detoxification.

62) Kasim, Manoefris, et al. "Improved myocardial perfusion in stable angina pectoris by oral lumbrokinase: a pilot study." The Journal of Alternative and Complementary Medicine 15.5 (2009): 539-544.

63) Paley, Mark R., and Pablo R. Ros. "Hepatic calcification." Radiologic Clinics 36.2 (1998): 391–398.

63) Aggarwal, Ramesh, Tauseef Akhthar, and Sachin Kumar Jain. "Coronary artery disease and its association with Vitamin D deficiency." Journal of mid-life health 7.2 (2016): 56.

64) Siadat, Zahra Dana, et al. "Association of vitamin D deficiency and coronary artery disease with cardiovascular risk factors." Journal of research in medical sciences: the official journal of Isfahan University of Medical Sciences 17.11 (2012): 1052.

65) Lee, Sunghee, et al. "A significant positive association of vitamin D deficiency with coronary artery calcification among middle-aged men: for the ERA JUMP study." Journal of the American College of Nutrition 35.7 (2016): 614–620.

66) Kukrele, P., and Ritesh Yadav. "Study of Vitamin D Level in Patient Presenting with Coronary Artery Disease."

67) Bamanikar, A. A., et al. "Prospective study of hypovitaminosis D in acute coronary syndrome." JMR 1.6 (2015): 163–166.

68) Dziedzic, Ewelina A., et al. "Association of Vitamin D Deficiency and Degree of Coronary Artery Disease in Cardiac Patients with Type 2 Diabetes." Journal of diabetes research 2017 (2017).

69) Wang, Chaoxun. "Role of vitamin d in cardiometabolic diseases." Experimental Diabetes Research 2013 (2013).

70) Kienreich, Katharina, et al. "Vitamin D and cardiovascular disease." Nutrients 5.8 (2013): 3005–3021.

71) Kumar, Y., and A. Bhatia. "Vitamin D and cardiovascular disease." Handbook of nutrition in heart health. Wageningen Academic Publishers, 2017. 213–220.

72) Moradi, Maryam, and Ali Foroutanfar. "evaluation of vitamin D levels in relation to coronary CT angiographic findings in an Iranian population." Vascular health and risk management 13 (2017): 361.

73) Wang, Thomas J., et al. "Vitamin D deficiency and risk of cardiovascular disease." Circulation 117.4 (2008): 503–511.

74) Watson, Karol E., et al. "Active serum vitamin D levels are inversely correlated with coronary calcification." Circulation 96.6 (1997): 1755–1760.

75) da Luz, P. L., et al. "Coronary artery plaque burden and calcium scores in healthy men adhering to long-term wine drinking or alcohol abstinence." Brazilian Journal of Medical and Biological Research 47.8 (2014):

76) Rao, Radhakrishna. "Endotoxemia and gut barrier dysfunction in alcoholic liver disease." Hepatology 50.2 (2009): 638–644.

77) Purohit, Vishnudutt, et al. "Alcohol, intestinal bacterial growth, intestinal permeability to endotoxin, and medical consequences: summary of a symposium." Alcohol 42.5 (2008): 349–361.

78) Keshavarzian, Ali, et al. "Evidence that chronic alcohol exposure promotes intestinal oxidative stress, intestinal hyperpermeability and endotoxemia prior to development of alcoholic steatohepatitis in rats." Journal of hepatology 50.3 (2009): 538–547.

79) Worthington, B. S., L. Meserole, and J. A. Syrotuck. "Effect of daily ethanol ingestion on intestinal permeability to macromolecules." The American journal of digestive diseases 23.1 (1978): 23.

80) Parlesak, Alexandr, et al. "Increased intestinal permeability to macromolecules and endotoxemia in patients with chronic alcohol abuse in different stages of alcohol-induced liver disease□." Journal of hepatology 32.5 (2000): 742–747.

81) Zhong, Wei, et al. "The role of zinc deficiency in alcohol-induced intestinal barrier dysfunction." American Journal of Physiology-Gastrointestinal and Liver Physiology 298.5 (2010): G625-G633.

82) Wang, Yuhua, et al. "Lactobacillus rhamnosus GG culture supernatant ameliorates acute alcohol-induced intestinal permeability and liver injury." American Journal of Physiology-Gastrointestinal and Liver Physiology 303.1 (2012): G32-G41.

83) Manco, Melania, Lorenza Putignani, and Gian Franco Bottazzo. "Gut microbiota, lipopolysaccharides, and innate immunity in the pathogenesis of obesity and cardiovascular risk." Endocrine reviews 31.6 (2010): 817–844.

86) Lee, Sang-Hong, et al. "Effect of Coronary Artery Calcification Score by Lifestyle and Correlation With Coronary Artery Stenosis by Multidetector Computed Tomography." Journal of computer assisted tomography 41.2 (2017): 236–241.

87) Maruthur, Nisa M., Nae-Yuh Wang, and Lawrence J. Appel. "Lifestyle interventions reduce coronary heart disease risk: results from the PREMIER Trial." Circulation 119.15 (2009): 2026–2031.

88) Lisspers, Jan, et al. "Long-term effects of lifestyle behavior change in coronary artery disease: effects on recurrent coronary events after percutaneous coronary intervention." Health Psychology 24.1 (2005): 41.

89) Kromhout, Daan, et al. "Prevention of coronary heart disease by diet and lifestyle: evidence from prospective cross-cultural, cohort, and intervention studies." Circulation 105.7 (2002): 893–898.

90) Ornish, Dean, et al. "Intensive lifestyle changes for reversal of coronary heart disease." Jama 280.23 (1998): 2001–2007.

91) Ornish, Dean, et al. "Can lifestyle changes reverse coronary heart disease?: The Lifestyle Heart Trial." The Lancet 336.8708 (1990): 129–133.

92) Jhamnani, Sunny, et al. "Meta-analysis of the effects of lifestyle modifications on coronary and carotid atherosclerotic burden." American Journal of Cardiology 115.2 (2015): 268–275.

93) Watts, G. F., et al. "Effects on coronary artery disease of lipid-lowering diet, or diet plus cholestyramine, in the St Thomas' Atherosclerosis Regression Study (STARS)." The Lancet 339.8793 (1992): 563–569.

94) Perrotta, Cristiana, et al. "The thyroid hormone triiodothyronine controls macrophage maturation and functions: protective role during inflammation." The American journal of pathology 184.1 (2014): 230–247.

CHAPTER
16

Thirty-Nine Reasons to Avoid
Bypass and Stenting

NO BOOK ON THE HEART would be complete without a discussion of invasive treatments offered by mainstream cardiology and cardiac surgery. This is the plumbing approach to the disease. The job of the invasive cardiologist is to find the clogged artery and then unclog it with a balloon angioplasty, stent, or surgical bypass graft, much the same as a plumber unclogs your drainpipe.

The Plumbing Approach

As we have seen, the pathologic process causing atherosclerosis is quite different from the clogged drainage pipe. The arteries are part of a living organism, with underlying cellular inflammation and calcification. Your arteries contain smooth muscle cells innervated by the autonomic nervous system. This controls vascular tone, the dilation or constriction of the vascular tree. Obviously, blood vessels are much more sophisticated than the plumbing pipe! And unlike your pipes, they are alive. In the same way, the plaque in our arteries is quite different from the debris and sediment clogging your kitchen drain. Perhaps these differences can explain the disappointing results with the "plumbing approach" to clogged arteries.

Progression of Atherosclerosis

The plumbing approach to cardiac disease fails to address the atherosclerotic disease process that continues after the procedure is completed. The procedure may be a success; however, progression of atherosclerosis may cause a recurrent heart attack.

Medical vs. Invasive Treatment for Coronary Artery Disease?

In this chapter, we will compare outcomes for invasive treatment versus medical treatment. Considering the hype and glory associated with cardiac procedures such as bypass and stenting, one might be surprised to find that their overall success rate is not much different than medical therapy with cardiac drugs.

Lucky for us, a large number of medical studies exist comparing invasive to conservative treatment with drugs. These studies reveal that invasive treatment with coronary bypass graft surgery or balloon angioplasty with stenting yield similar clinical outcomes to conservative medical treatment with cardiac drugs. It might surprise you that invasive treatment for the patient with stable angina provides about the same results as conservative medical treatment with cardiac drugs.

Brain Damage from Cardiac Bypass

Follow-up studies after cardiac bypass reveal that about half (50%) of patients having coronary bypass surgery suffer brain damage with permanent loss of memory and mental function from the procedure. (1–3) Obviously, this is not a good thing.

Although the medical literature suggests that optimal medical treatment (OMT) should initially be offered to the patient with stable angina, many times this is step is ignored, and the initial treatment offered may be a bypass or stent procedure. Based on the imagined or perceived urgency of the case, the patient may be persuaded to accept invasive rather than initial medical treatment. For the physicians, the financial rewards for the invasive procedure are considerably greater. Could this possibly play a role in the decision-making process?

Reduced Mortality with Cardiac Bypass

Coronary bypass operation reduces mortality in certain cases, such as a left main coronary artery lesion (the "widow-maker"), and in those cases with reduced left ventricular (LV) ejection fraction.(62) However, Dr. Eugene Caracciolo reports in 1995 in *Circulation* that no mortality benefit over and above medical treatment is obtained in surgical bypass of the left main lesion with normal LV ejection fraction. (62) In this case, the mortality benefit is similar to that of medical treatment.

Stent-Era Trials

Acute cardiac syndrome, also called myocardial infarction, is a special case in which invasive procedures are beneficial. Stenting after thrombolysis for acute myocardial Infarction reduces mortality. Dr. Bruno Scheller's 2003 study in Germany showed that immediate stenting after administering clot-dissolving drugs gave better mortality results when compared to delayed stenting. (79) Three more recent stent-era trials have shown favorable reduction in mortality with stenting. (80) However, this has not been consistently demonstrated. For multivessel coronary disease, no advantage over medical treatment was seen with coronary stenting. Dr. Richard Shemin, writing in 2008 in *Circulation* states:

> *Survival advantages of stent therapy for coronary artery disease over medical therapy have not been a consistent result in clinical trials. (60)*

Bypass Compared to Stenting

Compared to CABG (coronary artery bypass graft), there is no advantage for stenting. A five-year trial by Dr. Patrick Serruys published in 2005 comparing stenting to CABG for multivessel disease showed no difference in mortality outcome for the two groups, whether stented or bypassed. (82)

Here is a list of drugs used in medical treatment for coronary artery disease:

- Beta blockers such as Inderal
- Calcium-channel blockers include Cardizem, Procardia, and Norvasc.
- Nitrates such as Isordil, Sorbitrate, Cardilate, Dilatrate, and Peritrate. Nitroglycerine skin patches include Minitran, Nitro-Dur and Transderm-Nitro.
- Diuretics and ACE inhibitors
- Anti-platelet agents such as aspirin, dipyridamole, clopidogrel.
- Medical treatment includes propranolol, nifedipine, isosorbide dinitrate, dipyridamole and aspirin. (50)

Why Does Medical Therapy Work as Well as Invasive Procedures?

Medical therapy reduces the oxygen demand of the heart muscle and allows time for the heart to develop microscopic collateral vessels that provide blood flow around the blocked arteries.

A Randomized Trial

In 2004, Dr. W. Hueb reported his randomized trial comparing medical treatment to CABG (bypass), and percutaneous coronary intervention (PCI; intervention with balloon and stenting). (64) Six hundred and eleven patients with stable angina and angiographically documented double- or triple-vessel disease were randomly assigned to one of the three treatments, 1) medical treatment, 2) CABG or 3) PCI. Here are the results as quoted from the authors:

> Our results are consistent with the Coronary Artery Surgery Study (CASS) trial, in which no difference was seen between patients in the surgical and medical groups in terms of mortality, Q-wave MI, or event-free survival rates after five years of follow-up. In the CASS trial, a subgroup of patients with preserved ventricular function and mild stable angina was more likely to experience event-free survival with MT

[medical treatment] alone, even in the presence of three-vessel CAD [coronary artery disease]. (64)

The authors further state:

There were no significant differences among the cumulative cardiac-related mortality curves associated with the three therapeutic strategies. There were nine deaths in the PCI group, eight deaths in the CABG group, and three deaths in the MT group (p = 0.23). The cumulative survival rates at one year for patients assigned to each group were 96% for PCI, 96% for CABG, and 98% for MT." (64)

Dr. Evangelos Chatzistamatiou's 2011 report, "Stable Coronary Artery Disease: Latest Data in the Battle Between Conservative and Invasive Management," in the *Hellenic Journal of Cardiology* is an up-to-date summary listing indications for revascularization for stable angina patients. The authors conclude as follows:

In patients with chronic stable CAD, OMT (optimal medical therapy) is the first line treatment and should include all necessary ingredients in doses that can achieve the therapeutic goals. (71)

Orbita Placebo-Controlled Trial

The final nail is Rita Redberg's 2018 *Lancet* editorial on the ORBITA study, "*Last Nail in Coffin for PCI in Stable Angina?*" (84) The ORBITA study compared stenting to a sham procedure in a single coronary vessel otherwise medically treated. The study showed no difference in outcome for the stent vs. medical treatment. Dr. Redberg says:

The results of ORBITA show unequivocally that there are no benefits for PCI (stenting) compared with medical therapy for stable angina, even when angina is refractory to medical therapy. Based on these data, all cardiology guidelines should be revised to downgrade the recommendation for PCI in patients with angina despite use of medical therapy. (85)

Dr. David J Maron sums up the current state of the art as of April 2018:

Prior trials comparing a strategy of optimal medical therapy with or without revascularization have not shown that revascularization reduces cardiovascular events in patients with stable ischemic heart disease (SIHD) (86)

In summary, the decision to undergo cardiac bypass graft (CABG), with its long recovery time and adverse effect on neurocognitive function should not be taken lightly. With the exception of the left main coronary lesion (the widow maker) which is optimally treated with a revascularization procedure such as bypass or stent (83)(89), published studies support OMT as the first-line treatment for chronic stable angina.

♦ ♦ ♦ ♦ ♦

♦ References for Chapter 16

1) Longitudinal assessment of neurocognitive function after coronary artery bypass surgery. Newman MF1, et al. N Engl J Med. 2001 Feb 8;344(6):395–402.

2) Roach, Gary W., et al. "Adverse cerebral outcomes after coronary bypass surgery." New England Journal of Medicine 335.25 (1996): 1857–1864.

3) van Dijk, Diederik, et al. "Neurocognitive dysfunction after coronary artery bypass surgery: a systematic review." The Journal of Thoracic and Cardiovascular Surgery 120.4 (2000): 632–639.

4) 'Alternative' Medicine Is Mainstream. The evidence is mounting that diet and lifestyle are the best cures for our worst afflictions. By Deepak Chopra, Dean Ornish, Rustum Roy and Andrew Weil Jan. 9, 2009 Wall Street Journal Jan 2009

5) Boden, William E., et al. "Optimal medical therapy with or without PCI for stable coronary disease." New England Journal of Medicine 356.15 (2007): 1503–1516.

6) Angioplasty Fails Again and Again (8 out of 8 times) by John McDougal MD April 2000 Newsletter

7) Pursnani, Seema, et al. "Percutaneous Coronary Intervention Versus Optimal Medical Therapy in Stable Coronary Artery Disease A Systematic Review and Meta-Analysis of Randomized Clinical Trials." Circulation: Cardiovascular Interventions 5.4 (2012): 476–490.

8) Loder E. Curbing Medical Enthusiasm. BMJ 2007, April 7; 334:

9) Hochman JS, Coronary intervention for persistent occlusion after myocardial infarction. N Engl J Med. 2006 Dec 7;355(23):2395–407.

10) Hochman JS, Steg PG. Does preventive PCI work? N Engl J Med. 2007 Apr 12;356(15):1572–4.

11) Murphy, Marvin L., et al. "Treatment of chronic stable angina: a preliminary report of survival data of the randomized Veterans Administration Cooperative Study." New England Journal of Medicine 297.12 (1977): 621–627.

12) CASS Principal Investigators and Their Associates*. "Myocardial infarction and mortality in the coronary artery surgery study (CASS) randomized trial." New England Journal of Medicine 310.12 (1984): 750–758.

14) deleted

15) Wexler, Laura F., et al. "Non–Q-wave myocardial infarction following thrombolytic therapy: a comparison of outcomes in patients randomized to invasive or conservative post-infarct assessment strategies in the Veterans Affairs non–Q-wave Infarction Strategies In-Hospital (VANQWISH) trial." Journal of the American College of Cardiology 37.1 (2001): 19–25.

16) Bucher, Heiner C., et al. "Percutaneous transluminal coronary angioplasty versus medical treatment for non-acute coronary heart disease: meta-analysis of randomised controlled trials." Bmj 321.7253 (2000): 73–77.

17) Wallentin, Lars, et al. "Outcome at 1 year after an invasive compared with a non-invasive strategy in unstable coronary-artery disease: the FRISC II invasive randomised trial." The Lancet 356.9223 (2000): 9–16.

18) Lagerqvist, Bo, et al. "5-year outcomes in the FRISC-II randomised trial of an invasive versus a non-invasive strategy in non-ST-elevation acute coronary syndrome: a follow-up study." The Lancet 368.9540 (2006): 998–1004.

19) Dakik, Habib A., et al. "Intensive medical therapy versus coronary angioplasty for suppression of myocardial ischemia in survivors of acute myocardial infarction: a prospective, randomized pilot study." Circulation 98.19 (1998): 2017–2023.

20) Pflieger, Matthew, et al. "Medical management of stable coronary artery disease." American family physician 83.7 (2011): 819–826.

21) Boden, William E. "Medical Management of Stable Coronary Artery Disease." Evidence-Based Cardiology, Third Edition: 343–356.

22) Boden, William E., et al. "Outcomes in patients with acute non–Q-wave myocardial infarction randomly assigned to an invasive as compared with a conservative management strategy." New England Journal of Medicine 338.25 (1998): 1785–1792.

23) Peduzzi, Peter, Ayumi Kamina, and Katherine Detre. "Twenty-two-year follow-up in the VA cooperative study of coronary artery bypass surgery for stable angina." American Journal of Cardiology 81.12 (1998): 1393–1399.

24) McCullough, Peter A., et al. "A prospective randomized trial of triage angiography in acute coronary syndromes ineligible for thrombolytic therapy: results of the Medicine versus Angiography in Thrombolytic Exclusion (MATE) trial." Journal of the American College of Cardiology 32.3 (1998): 596–605.

25) Madsen, Jan K., et al. "Danish multicenter randomized study of invasive versus conservative treatment in patients with inducible ischemia after thrombolysis in acute myocardial infarction (DANAMI)." Circulation 96.3 (1997): 748–755.

26) Chamberlain, D. A., et al. "Coronary angioplasty versus medical therapy for angina: the second Randomised Intervention Treatment of Angina (RITA-2) trial." The Lancet 350.9076 (1997): 461.

27) Henderson, Robert A., et al. "Seven-year outcome in the RITA-2 trial: coronary angioplasty versus medical therapy." Journal of the American College of Cardiology 42.7 (2003): 1161–1170.

28) Anderson, H. Vernon, et al. "One-year results of the Thrombolysis in Myocardial Infarction (TIMI) IIIB clinical trial: a randomized comparison of tissue-type plasminogen activator versus placebo and early invasive versus early conservative strategies in unstable angina and non-Q wave myocardial infarction." Journal of the American College of Cardiology 26.7 (1995): 1643–1650.

29) Hueb, Whady A., et al. "The Medicine, Angioplasty or Surgery Study (MASS): a prospective, randomized trial of medical therapy, balloon angioplasty or bypass surgery for single proximal left anterior descending artery stenoses." Journal of the American College of Cardiology 26.7 (1995): 1600–1605.

30) Hueb, Whady, et al. "Five-year follow-up of the Medicine, Angioplasty, or Surgery Study (MASS II): a randomized controlled clinical trial of 3 therapeutic strategies for multivessel coronary artery disease." Circulation 115.9 (2007): 1082–1089.

31) TIMI IIIb Investigators. "Effects of tissue plasminogen activator and a comparison of early invasive and conservative strategies in unstable angina and non-Q-wave myocardial infarction: results of the TIMI IIIB trial." Circulation 89.4 (1994): 1545–1556.

32) Terrin, Michael L., et al. "Two-and three-year results of the thrombolysis in myocardial infraction (TIMI) phase II clinical trial." Journal of the American College of Cardiology 22.7 (1993): 1763–1772.

34) Ellis, Stephen G., et al. "Randomized trial of late elective angioplasty versus conservative management for patients with residual stenoses after thrombolytic treatment of myocardial infarction. Treatment of Post-Thrombolytic Stenoses (TOPS) Study Group." Circulation 86.5 (1992): 1400–1406.

35) Parisi, Alfred F., Edward D. Folland, and Pamela Hartigan. "A comparison of angioplasty with medical therapy in the treatment of single-vessel coronary artery disease." New England Journal of Medicine 326.1 (1992): 10–16.

36) SWIFT (Should We Intervene Following Thrombolysis?) Trial Study Group. "SWIFT trial of delayed elective intervention v conservative treatment after thrombolysis with anistreplase in acute myocardial infarction." BMJ: British Medical Journal (1991): 555–560.

37) Rogers, William J., et al. "Comparison of immediate invasive, delayed invasive, and conservative strategies after tissue-type plasminogen activator. Results of the Thrombolysis in Myocardial Infarction (TIMI) Phase II-A trial." Circulation 81.5 (1990): 1457–1476.

38) Barbash, Gabriel I., et al. "Randomized controlled trial of late in-hospital angiography and angioplasty versus conservative management after treatment with recombinant tissue-type plasminogen activator in acute myocardial infarction." The American journal of cardiology 66.5 (1990): 538–545.

39) TIMI Study Group*. "Comparison of invasive and conservative strategies after treatment with intravenous tissue plasminogen activator in acute myocardial infarction." New England Journal of Medicine 320.10 (1989): 618–627.

40) Simoons, M. L., et al. "Thrombolysis with tissue plasminogen activator in acute myocardial infarction: no additional benefit from immediate percutaneous coronary angioplasty." The Lancet 331.8579 (1988): 197–203.

41) Luchi, Robert J., et al. "Comparison of medical and surgical treatment for unstable angina pectoris." New England Journal of Medicine 316.16 (1987): 977–984.

43) MAHRER, Peter R. "Outcome study of two large populations with different rates of cardiac interventions." Cardiovascular reviews & reports 21.12 (2000): 638–651.

44) Piegas, Leopoldo S., et al. "The Organization to Assess Strategies for Ischemic Syndromes (OASIS) registry in patients with unstable angina." The American journal of cardiology 84.5 (1999): 7–12.

45) Tu, Jack V., et al. "Use of cardiac procedures and outcomes in elderly patients with myocardial infarction in the United States and Canada." New England Journal of Medicine 336.21 (1997): 1500–1505.

46) McGovern, Paul G., et al. "Comparison of medical care and one-and
12-month mortality of hospitalized patients with acute myocardial infarction
in Minneapolis-St. Paul, Minnesota, United States of America and Göteborg,
Sweden." American Journal of Cardiology 80.5 (1997): 557–562.

48) Van Norman, Gail A., and Karen Posner. "Coronary stenting or percutaneous
transluminal coronary angioplasty prior to noncardiac surgery increases adverse
perioperative cardiac events: the evidence is mounting." Journal of the American
College of Cardiology 36.7 (2000): 2351.

49) Kałuza, Grzegorz L., et al. "Catastrophic outcomes of noncardiac surgery soon
after coronary stenting." Journal of the American College of Cardiology 35.5
(2000): 1288–1294.

50) Hueb, Whady, et al. "Two-to eight-year survival rates in patients who refused
coronary artery bypass grafting." The American journal of cardiology 63.3
(1989): 155–159..

51) Prognosis of Medically Treated Patients with Coronary Artery Disease With
Profound ST-Segment Depression During Exercise Testing. Podrif, PD,
Graboys, TB, Lown, B. N Engl J Med. 1981; 305:1111–1116.

52) Thompson, Craig A., et al. "Exercise performance-based outcomes of medically
treated patients with coronary artery disease and profound ST segment
depression." Journal of the American College of Cardiology 36.7 (2000):
2140–2145.

53) Katritsis, Demosthenes G., and John PA Ioannidis. "Percutaneous coronary
intervention versus conservative therapy in nonacute coronary artery disease: a
meta-analysis." Circulation 111.22 (2005): 2906–2912.

54) Beck, Christine A., Mark J. Eisenberg, and Louise Pilote. "Invasive versus
noninvasive management of ST-elevation acute myocardial infarction: a review
of clinical trials and observational studies." American heart journal 149.2 (2005):
194–199.

55) Wijeysundera, Harindra C., et al. "An early invasive strategy versus ischemia-
guided management after fibrinolytic therapy for ST-segment elevation
myocardial infarction: a meta-analysis of contemporary randomized controlled
trials." American heart journal 156.3 (2008): 564–572.

56) Cantor, Warren J., et al. "Immediate angioplasty after thrombolysis: a systematic
review." Canadian Medical Association Journal 173.12 (2005): 1473–1481.

57) Scheller, Bruno, et al. "Beneficial effects of immediate stenting after thrombolysis in acute myocardial infarction." Journal of the American College of Cardiology 42.4 (2003): 634–641.

58) VA Coronary Artery Bypass Surgery Cooperative Study Group. "Eighteen-year follow-up in the Veterans Affairs Cooperative Study of Coronary Artery Bypass Surgery for stable angina." Circulation 86.1 (1992): 121.

59) deleted

60) Shemin, Richard J. "Coronary artery bypass grafting versus stenting for unprotected left main coronary artery disease: where lies the body of proof?." (2008): 2326–2329.

61) Serruys, Patrick W., et al. "Five-year outcomes after coronary stenting versus bypass surgery for the treatment of multivessel disease: the final analysis of the Arterial Revascularization Therapies Study (ARTS) randomized trial." Journal of the American College of Cardiology 46.4 (2005): 575–581.

62) Caracciolo, Eugene A., et al. "Comparison of surgical and medical group survival in patients with left main coronary artery disease long-term CASS experience." Circulation 91.9 (1995): 2325–2334.

63) Boden, William E. "Surgery, angioplasty, or medical therapy for symptomatic multivessel coronary artery disease: Is there an indisputable "winning strategy" from evidence-based clinical trials?." Journal of the American College of Cardiology 43.10 (2004): 1752–1754.

64) Hueb, Whady, et al. "The medicine, angioplasty, or surgery study (MASS-II): a randomized, controlled clinical trial of three therapeutic strategies for multivessel coronary artery disease: one-year results." Journal of the American College of Cardiology 43.10 (2004): 1743–1751.

65) Hueb, Whady, et al. "Ten-year follow-up survival of the Medicine, Angioplasty, or Surgery Study (MASS II): a randomized controlled clinical trial of 3 therapeutic strategies for multivessel coronary artery disease." Circulation 122.10 (2010): 949-957.

66) Williams DO, Vasaiwala SC, Boden WE. Is optimal medical therapy "optimal therapy" for multivessel coronary artery disease? Optimal management of multivessel coronary artery disease. Circulation. 2010;122:943–945.

67) Manché, Alexander. " optimal treatment multivessel coronary artery disease " (2014).

68) Smith, Peter K. "Treatment selection for coronary artery disease: the collision of a belief system with evidence." The Annals of thoracic surgery 87.5 (2009): 1328–1331.

69) IZQUIERDA, ARTERIA CORONARIA, CORONARY ARTERY-BYPASS GRAFT OR PERCUTANEOUS CORONARY INTERVENTION FOR LEFT MAIN CORONARY ARTERY LESIONS: AN ONGOING DISCUSSION." CorSalud 2012 Oct-Dec;4(4):228–231

70) ElGuindy, Ahmed M., and Ahmed Afifi. "PCI versus CABG in patients with complex coronary artery disease: Time for reconciliation?." Global cardiology science & practice 2012.2 (2012): 18.

71) CHATZISTAMATIOU, EVANGELOS I., et al. "Stable Coronary Artery Disease: Latest Data in the Battle Between Conservative and Invasive Management." Hellenic J Cardiol 52 (2011): 516–524.

72) Bypassing Bypass Surgery by Elmer M. Cranton, M.D.

73) Peduzzi, Peter, Ayumi Kamina, and Katherine Detre. "Twenty-two-year follow-up in the VA cooperative study of coronary artery bypass surgery for stable angina." American Journal of Cardiology 81.12 (1998): 1393–1399.

74) Deedwania, Prakash C., and Enrique V. Carbajal. "Medical therapy versus myocardial revascularization in chronic coronary syndrome and stable angina." The American journal of medicine 124.8 (2011): 681–688.

75) Chatterjee, Debjit. "Medical management of angina: treatment of associated conditions and the role of antiplatelet drugs." Vol. 15, N° 10 – 12 Jul 2017 European Society of Cardiology Journals E-Journal of Cardiology Practice Volume 15

76) Ranganatha, M., et al. "Medical management and evaluations of stable angina patients in tertiary care centre without invasive treatment." International Journal of Advances in Medicine 4.5 (2017): 1260–1265.

77) Pflieger, Matthew, et al. "Medical management of stable coronary artery disease." American family physician 83.7 (2011).

78) Sawhney, J. P. S., et al. "The role of optimal medical therapy in patients with stable coronary artery disease." Journal of Clinical and Preventive Cardiology 7.2 (2018): 60.

79) Scheller, Bruno, et al. "Beneficial effects of immediate stenting after thrombolysis in acute myocardial infarction." Journal of the American College of Cardiology 42.4 (2003): 634–641.

80) Cantor, Warren J., et al. "Immediate angioplasty after thrombolysis: a systematic review." Canadian Medical Association Journal 173.12 (2005): 1473–1481.

81) deleted

82) Serruys, Patrick W., et al. "Five-year outcomes after coronary stenting versus bypass surgery for the treatment of multivessel disease: the final analysis of the Arterial Revascularization Therapies Study (ARTS) randomized trial." Journal of the American College of Cardiology 46.4 (2005): 575–581.

83) Takaro, Timothy, et al. "The VA cooperative randomized study of surgery for coronary arterial occlusive disease II. Subgroup with significant left main lesions." Circulation 54.6 Suppl (1976): III107–17.

84) Brown, David L., and Rita F. Redberg. "Last nail in the coffin for PCI in stable angina?." The Lancet 391.10115 (2018): 3–4.

85) Al-Lamee, Rasha, et al. "Percutaneous coronary intervention in stable angina (ORBITA): a double-blind, randomised controlled trial." The Lancet 391.10115 (2018): 31–40.

86) Maron, David J., et al. "International Study of Comparative Health Effectiveness with Medical and Invasive Approaches (ISCHEMIA) Trial: Rationale and Design." American Heart Journal (2018).

87) BARI 2D Study Group. "A randomized trial of therapies for type 2 diabetes and coronary artery disease." New England Journal of Medicine 360.24 (2009): 2503–2515.

88) Furtado, Mariana Vargas, et al. "Effectiveness of Medical and Revascularization Procedures as the Initial Strategy in Stable Coronary Artery Disease: A Cohort Study." International Journal of Cardiovascular Sciences 30.5 (2017): 408–415.

89) Holmes Jr, David R., and Malcolm R. Bell. "Left anterior descending artery stenosis: the widow maker revisited." Mayo Clinic Proceedings. Vol. 75. No. 11. Elsevier, 2000.

Atherosclerosis: How Does it Happen?

ATHEROSCLEROTIC PLAQUE FORMATION IS A series of events. The first event is the deposit of lipoproteins, called the "fatty streak," which eventually becomes the lipid core of the plaque. We know the fatty streak is the first step because it has been observed in the human fetus. (18) Now, that's really early! The next step in plaque formation is infiltration with cells called monocytes. Dr. Mohamad Navab from UCLA published an excellent review of the mechanism of atherosclerotic plaque formation. (2)

The Linus Pauling Theory, Vitamin C Deficiency, and Cholesterol Patches

Linus Pauling and others suspected that the depositing of LDL cholesterol in the wall serves as patching material to repair small cracks in the arterial wall at sites of mechanical stress from pulsations and flow turbulence. Pauling theorized that, because of a subclinical vitamin C deficiency, the normal repair mechanisms are ineffective, so that an alternate repair mechanism with LDL cholesterol evolved. The LDL cholesterol serves as a sort of rubber cement to patch up the cracks in arteries, just we as patch the inner tube of a tire.

Since the fatty streak appears so early in life, at the fetal stage, it is likely there is a constant ebb and flow of lipoprotein material in and out of the arterial wall. We now know there is a transport mechanism, in the form of LDL particles, for cholesterol to travel in the bloodstream to the arterial wall. There is also a reverse cholesterol transport mechanism that transports cholesterol back from the artery wall to the liver in the form of HDL particles using the LCAT enzyme (lecithin cholesterol acetyl transferase).

Cholesterol Transport: Good (HDL) and Bad (LDL) Cholesterol

The LDL particles are transported from the liver in the bloodstream out to the body tissues, where cholesterol is delivered to the fatty streak in the artery wall. The HDL particles carry cholesterol from the fatty streak in the artery wall back to the liver, where it is metabolized and excreted as bile. Thus LDL is "bad" and HDL is "good." (4)

Oxidized Cholesterol

The reality is that LDL cholesterol itself is not the culprit; rather, it is oxidized LDL that is the "bad guy." Lowering plain LDL cholesterol will also lower the oxidized fraction of LDL cholesterol, but this is a rather crude way to do it. Cholesterol is a building block for membranes and sex steroids that is important for overall health, and lower cholesterol is associated with increased mortality from cancer, liver disease, and mental disease. (5)(6) Cholesterol defends our body against LPS and low-level endotoxemia.

Perhaps this is the reason that, while lowering cholesterol with statin drugs can reduce "cardiac events," statin drugs, sadly, have little or no benefit in terms of all-cause mortality. It would be much more beneficial to selectively reduce only the OXIDIZED LDL cholesterol.

Researchers have tests to measure oxidized LDL cholesterol, but they are not yet widely available to clinicians. To remedy this, the major labs are quickly moving to add oxidized LDL as a routine lab test over the next few years.

The Role of Antioxidants

Selectively reducing oxidized LDL is exactly what is done by antioxidants like vitamin C, E, carotenoids, and polyphenol bioflavonoids. These dietary supplements, as well as a healthy diet and lifestyle, are clearly beneficial. (9) However, many people are confused by the opposing views in the medical literature and the media. These views oppose the use of dietary supplements to prevent heart disease. Some have even proposed the bizarre notion that vitamins increase mortality. Of course, these views represent the interests of the pharmaceutical industry, which stands to lose billions from a reduction in heart disease and a reduced demand for drugs. (10–14) It is clear that dietary antioxidants like carotenoids in fresh vegetables as well as resveratrol from red wine polyphenols inhibit LDL oxidation and reduce heart disease. (15) We will later look at novel antioxidants such as liposomal glutathione and Boswellia. (16)

Infiltration by Monocytes: Macrophages and Inflammation

The next step in plaque formation is the infiltration of cells into the wall of the artery. Current thinking is that oxidized LDL attracts the influx of mono-cytes. These are cells in the bloodstream which have the ability to transform themselves into large scavenger cells called macrophages which serve as the garbage trucks for pickup and disposal. They engulf, digest, and dispose of the old or toxic stuff the body needs to get rid of. These macrophages engulf the LDL cholesterol and try to dispose of it. But during the disposal process, more of the LDL is oxidized. Something goes wrong at this step, and the macrophages continue to accumulate more and more oxidized LDL until the poor cell looks like an overinflated balloon ready to burst. This becomes the "foam cell."

The Foam Cell: The Culprit is Oxidized LDL

This new overstuffed macrophage is now called a "foam cell" because it looks foamy under the microscope. It is clear that the culprit is the oxidized or rancid form of LDL cholesterol. If the LDL is not oxidized, there seems to be no problem, and the LDL can be transported out of the artery back to the liver in the form of HDL using the LCAT enzyme for reverse cholesterol transport.

The foam cells, however, accumulate and send out more chemical messages, which invoke an inflammatory cascade that attracts more macrophages and other cells in an inflammatory reaction. This inflammation in the wall of the artery causes the thickening in the wall called plaque formation.

The Fibrous Cap

The last step in plaque formation is the fibrous cap which seals the small puddle of oxidized LDL, macrophages and and inflammatory cells within the plaque, safely walling off the plaque from the flowing blood within the arterial lumen. Rupture of the fibrous cap is the event that exposes the thrombogenic plaque to the bloodstream, causing clot formation and heart attack.

How to Prevent Oxidation of LDL cholesterol

Now that we know the events leading to plaque formation and rupture, we can create a logical plan to prevent and reverse this process. Even after LDL becomes oxidized, it can be converted back to its original form with the use of antioxidants in a process called reduction. A number of antioxidants have been shown to be effective. The most important and most powerful intracellular antioxidant is glutathione, a simple structure composed of three amino acids and sulfur.

What is Glutathione?

Glutathione is the most powerful naturally occurring antioxidant in all human cells. It is a small simple compound composed of three amino acids, glutamic acid, cysteine, and glycine. Cysteine contains sulfur, accounting for its sulfur taste and smell.

Glutathione is found in all cells in the body, with the highest concentration in the liver, where it is important for detoxification and the elimination of toxins and products of oxidation called free radicals.

Liposomal Glutathione Reduces Plaque by 30%

A 2007 publication from the Technion in Haifa showed that liposomal glutathione reduced plaque formation by 30% in genetically modified ApoE mice. (16) These are mice that have accelerated atherosclerosis. The authors also found that glutathione peroxidase, the enzyme that allows the glutathione to refresh the oxidized LDL back to its original reduced form, is present in the LDL particle itself. How convenient to have this enzyme already in place on the LDL particle.

What is Boswellia ?

Oxidation of the LDL cholesterol involves the lipoxygenase pathway, which can be inhibited by an old botanical called Boswellia. Boswellia works as anti-inflammatory agent by inhibiting 5-lipoxygenase (5 LOX) and byproducts called leukotrienes. This pathway is important in chronic inflammatory diseases such as arthritis, colitis, asthma, allergies, osteoporosis, eczema, and psoriasis. Boswellia is also useful in preventing the inflammation inside the arterial tree associated with atherosclerotic plaque formation. In mice genetically altered so that they do not have 5-lipoxygenase, there is a 26-fold reduction in atherosclerotic plaque compared to controls. (17)

Currently, mainstream medicine has no drug to control the 5-LOX enzyme, because up to now the pharmaceutical industry has not been able to make such a drug without major adverse side effects.

However, Boswellia is a safe, natural, gum resin of the frankincense tree, which powerfully suppresses the 5-lipoxygenase enzyme like no other substance known. Ancient traditional uses and more recent studies have shown significant improvements in asthma, arthritis, colitis, allergies, and heart disease. The most active frankincense component is acetyl-11-keto-beta-boswellic acid (AKBA).

In a 2008 study, Dr. Cuaz-Pérolin studied the anti-inflammatory and anti-atherogenic effects of Boswellia in LPS-challenged ApoE mice. (1) Atherosclerotic lesions were induced by weekly LPS injections in ApoE mice. LPS injection into the mice more than doubled atherosclerotic lesion size. Treatment with AKBA Boswellia significantly reduced lesion size by more than 50%. (1)

Summary

The above description of the mechanics of atherosclerotic process is incomplete, as it contains no mention of the recent discovery of multiple micro-organisms within the plaque material. Nonetheless, interventions that reduce oxidized LDL, as shown with various botanical agents, may prove useful.

♦　♦　♦　♦　♦

◆ References for Chapter 17

1) Cuaz-Pérolin, Clarisse, et al. "Antiinflammatory and antiatherogenic effects of the NF-κB inhibitor acetyl-11-keto-β-boswellic acid in LPS-challenged ApoE−/− mice." Arteriosclerosis, thrombosis, and vascular biology 28.2 (2008): 272–277.

2) Navab, Mohamad, et al. "Thematic review series: the pathogenesis of atherosclerosis the oxidation hypothesis of atherogenesis: the role of oxidized phospholipids and HDL." Journal of lipid research 45.6 (2004): 993–1007.

3) Stocker, Roland, and John F. Keaney Jr. "Role of oxidative modifications in atherosclerosis." Physiological reviews 84.4 (2004): 1381–1478.

4) Colpo, Anthony. "LDL Cholesterol:" Bad" Cholesterol or Bad Science?." Journal of American Physicians and Surgeons 10.3 (2005): 83.

5) Shor, Renana, et al. "Low serum LDL cholesterol levels and the risk of fever, sepsis, and malignancy." Annals of Clinical & Laboratory Science 37.4 (2007): 343–348.

6) Ulmer, Hanno, et al. "Why Eve is not Adam: prospective follow-up in 149,650 women and men of cholesterol and other risk factors related to cardiovascular and all-cause mortality." Journal of Women's Health 13.1 (2004): 41–53.

7–8) deleted

9) Salonen, Riitta M., et al. "Six-year effect of combined vitamin C and E supplementation on atherosclerotic progression: the Antioxidant Supplementation in Atherosclerosis Prevention (ASAP) Study." Circulation 107.7 (2003): 947–953.

10) McCormick, Donald B. "The dubious use of vitamin-mineral supplements in relation to cardiovascular disease." The American journal of clinical nutrition 84.4 (2006): 680–681.

11) Elboudwarej, Omeed. "Vitamin C and Treating Coronary Artery Disease: More Hype than Hope?." Nutrition Bytes 14.1 (2010).

12) Hickey, Steve, Len Noriegai, and Hilary Roberts. "Poor methodology in meta-analysis of vitamins." Journal of Orthomolecular Medicine 22.1 (2007): 8.

13) Traber, Maret G. "Heart disease and single-vitamin supplementation−." The American journal of clinical nutrition 85.1 (2007): 293S-299S.

14) Hathcock, John N., et al. "Vitamins E and C are safe across a broad range of intakes." The American journal of clinical nutrition 81.4 (2005): 736–745.

15) Aviram, M., et al. "Dietary antioxidants and paraoxonases against LDL oxidation and atherosclerosis development." Atherosclerosis: Diet and Drugs. Springer, Berlin, Heidelberg, 2005. 263–300.

16) Rosenblat, Mira, et al. "Anti-oxidant and anti-atherogenic properties of liposomal glutathione: studies in vitro, and in the atherosclerotic apolipoprotein E-deficient mice." Atherosclerosis 195.2 (2007): e61-e68.

17) Mehrabian, Margarete, et al. "Identification of 5-lipoxygenase as a major gene contributing to atherosclerosis susceptibility in mice." Circulation research 91.2 (2002): 120–126.

18) Napoli, Claudio, et al. "Fatty streak formation occurs in human fetal aortas and is greatly enhanced by maternal hypercholesterolemia. Intimal accumulation of low density lipoprotein and its oxidation precede monocyte recruitment into early atherosclerotic lesions." The Journal of clinical investigation 100.11 (1997): 2680–2690.

19) Staprans, Ilona, et al. "Oxidized cholesterol in the diet accelerates the development of atherosclerosis in LDL receptor–and apolipoprotein E-deficient mice." Arteriosclerosis, thrombosis, and vascular biology 20.3 (2000): 708–714.

20) Staprans, Ilona, et al. "Oxidized cholesterol in the diet accelerates the development of aortic atherosclerosis in cholesterol-fed rabbits." Arteriosclerosis, thrombosis, and vascular biology 18.6 (1998): 977–983.

21) Mertens, A. N. N., and Paul Holvoet. "Oxidized LDL and HDL: antagonists in atherothrombosis." The FASEB journal 15.12 (2001): 2073–2084.

22) Shashkin, Pavel, Bojan Dragulev, and Klaus Ley. "Macrophage differentiation to foam cells." Current pharmaceutical design 11.23 (2005): 3061–3072.

23) deleted

24) Hayden, John M., et al. "Induction of monocyte differentiation and foam cell formation in vitro by 7-ketocholesterol." Journal of lipid research 43.1 (2002): 26–35.

25) Meisinger, Christa, et al. "Plasma oxidized low-density lipoprotein, a strong predictor for acute coronary heart disease events in apparently healthy, middle-aged men from the general population." Circulation 112.5 (2005): 651–657.

26) Wallenfeldt, K., et al. "Oxidized low-density lipoprotein in plasma is a prognostic marker of subclinical atherosclerosis development in clinically healthy men." Journal of internal medicine 256.5 (2004): 413–420.

27) Holvoet, Paul, et al. "The metabolic syndrome, circulating oxidized LDL, and risk of myocardial infarction in well-functioning elderly people in the health, aging, and body composition cohort." Diabetes 53.4 (2004): 1068–1073.

28) Rosenson-Schloss, Rene S., et al. "Glutathione Preconditioning Attenuates Ac-LDL–Induced Macrophage Apoptosis via Protein Kinase C–Dependent Ac-LDL Trafficking." Experimental Biology and Medicine 230.1 (2005): 40–48.

29) Blankenberg, Stefan, et al. "Glutathione peroxidase 1 activity and cardiovascular events in patients with coronary artery disease." New England Journal of Medicine 349.17 (2003): 1605–1613.

30) Ashfaq, Salman, et al. "The relationship between plasma levels of oxidized and reduced thiols and early atherosclerosis in healthy adults." Journal of the American College of Cardiology 47.5 (2006): 1005–1011.

31) Morrison, John A., et al. "Serum glutathione in adolescent males predicts parental coronary heart disease." Circulation 100.22 (1999): 2244–2247.

32) Prasad A, Andrews NP, Padder FA, et al. Glutathione reverses endothelial dysfunction and improves nitric oxide bioavailability. J Am Coll Cardiol 1999;34:507–514.

Preventing Heart Attacks with Ouabain

IN THE PREVIOUS CHAPTER, WE made the case for the "clogged artery" filled with atherosclerotic plaque as the cause for heart attacks. Indeed, imaging and autopsy studies show extensive arterial plaque formation in the unfortunate victims of heart attacks.

The Plumbing Approach to Heart Disease

Recognizing the "clogged artery" as the cause of heart attacks, an entire medical industry is busy unclogging arteries with the "plumbing approach." This was my job during my years working as an interventional radiologist. I was one of the doctors serving as glorified plumbers, advancing catheters, angioplasty balloons, and stents into the patient to open up these clogged arteries. If the catheters, balloons, and stents fail, the operating room is next—the cardiac bypass operation. Those patients who manage to avoid the invasive cardiologist may be given "medical treatment" with cardiac drugs such as statins, beta blockers, calcium-channel blockers, nitrates, aspirin, blood thinners, and so on.

What Causes Heart Attacks?

According to mainstream cardiology, heart attacks are caused by obstruction of the coronary artery shutting off oxygen supply to a segment of the heart muscle, which then undergoes "infarction," a word meaning cell death from lack of oxygen. No doubt this does happen in most but not all cases.

Heart Attack with Normal Coronary Arteries, Clogged Arteries with No Heart Attack

You might be surprised to know that about 1 to 12% of heart attacks can occur with completely normal coronary arteries, as demonstrated by angiography or autopsy examination. (41) (25–31). Not only that, autopsy studies on young trauma victims show left main coronary artery or multivessel disease in 20% of cases, placing them at high risk, yet heart attacks are rare in this age group. (42)

Autopsy Studies

Autopsy studies of hospitalized patients who die of non-cardiac causes show that 41.6% have critical stenosis or occlusion of at least one major vessel. (43) You might ask the obvious question. Why didn't these patients die from heart attack instead of the non-cardiac cause? Clearly there must be other factors at work. Clogged arteries are quite common, and some people seem to survive in spite of it. We will pick up this idea later.

Coronary Artery Theory

In the "Coronary Artery Theory of Heart Attacks," the arterial plaque continues to enlarge, causing narrowing of the arterial lumen (also called stenosis). This stenosis is like closing a water faucet, reducing blood flow down to a trickle. Finally, the "ruptured plaque" is the end-stage event triggering thrombosis and total obstruction of the coronary artery. Downstream from the blocked artery, the myocardial muscle segment undergoes cell death from lack of oxygen. This is called a myocardial infarction, or heart attack.

The CABG-Zipper Club

This Coronary Artery Theory is the working hypothesis for all invasive cardiologists who never question it and happily go about their job as glorified plumbers, searching out all the clogged arteries and unclogging them in the cardiac cath lab. Their job is to inject radiographic dye into the coronary arteries looking for the stenosis. If a severely narrowed artery is discovered, the invasive cardiologist will promptly perform a plumbing procedure—the angioplasty or stent to open the narrowed artery. If this proves unsuccessful, the patient may then go next door to the surgical suite to undergo a coronary artery bypass graft. A massive medical industry has been built on the Coronary Artery Theory of heart disease. Your local hospital might very well be in an expansion phase, building larger facilities to do all this.

How to Reduce Atherosclerotic Plaque with Diet and Lifestyle

Obviously, atherosclerosis is a bad thing. How do we prevent it? How do we halt progression of all these atherosclerotic plaques in our arteries? Chapter 16 explains our program for slowing progression of calcium score with OMT, diet, and lifestyle modification. The annual calcium score test is our tool for determining rate of progression of disease, as well as response to diet and lifestyle modification.

A Differing Viewpoint: The Plumbers Are Wrong

In a May 2014 article, Dr. Thomas Cowan proposed an alternate theory of heart attacks called the "Myogenic Theory." (1) Although arterial plaque is a bad thing, Dr. Cowan says the "plumbing" approach to clogged arteries is a futile exercise. In agreement with Dr. Cowan is Dr. Howard H. Wayne, who says most studies show no benefit for "plumbing procedures" compared to OMT.

The 2003 Mayo Clinic Study

A representative study is the large 2003 Mayo Clinic study, which concludes that cardiac bypass relieves chest pain but does not prevent further heart attacks, and that only high-risk patients whose lives are in acute danger benefit from cardiac surgery. (36)

MASS II Study

Another representative study is the MASS II by Dr. Hueb published in *Circulation* in 2007. Dr. Hueb says outcomes for cardiac bypass and stenting are about the same as medical therapy (with drugs) for multivessel coronary artery disease with stable angina and good left-ventricular ejection fraction:

Despite routine use of coronary artery bypass graft (CABG) and percutaneous coronary intervention (PCI), no conclusive evidence exists that either modality is superior to medical therapy (MT) alone for treating multivessel coronary artery disease with stable angina and preserved ventricular function.

All three treatment regimens yielded comparable, relatively low rates of death. Medical Therapy was associated with an incidence of long-term events and rate of additional revascularization similar to those for Percutaneous Coronary Intervention (balloon and stent). (44)

Courage Study: "The Plumbers" vs. "the Pill Pushers"

The Courage Study, which is one of Dr. Cowan's favorites, found no mortality benefit for percutaneous angioplasty compared to medical treatment alone in patients with stable coronary artery disease (stable ischemic heart disease—that is, the patient was not having an acute heart attack at the time of presentation). (33–34) Only the "high risk" patient, or patient with acute heart attack at time of presentation benefits from revascularization with angioplasty or bypass with improved survival (a mortality benefit). (35,36) Here, the ability to differentiate between stable heart disease and "high-risk heart disease" becomes important.

Problems with the Plumbing Approach

As we see from numerous published studies, the "plumbing approach" to coronary artery disease with stents and bypass operations has been a disappointment, with no reduction in mortality compared to medical treatment for the patient with chronic stable angina. However, there is a plumbing benefit, as mentioned above, for the high-risk patient. We will now look into this to find out why. (35,36)

With the exception of the bypass or stent for the "high risk patient," that is, someone with a left main coronary artery lesion, also known as the "widow maker," cardiac "plumbing" procedures have been a disappointment. In the stable angina patient, benefits of plumbing procedures are about the same as medical treatment. (45) Why is that?

Formation of Collateral Circulation: A Quick Trip to the Dog Lab

A 1976 study in *Circulation* by Dr. W. Schaper, working in the dog lab, is illustrative. (46) When the dog's coronary artery is suddenly occluded, the dog suffers a heart attack and could die. However, if the dog's coronary artery is *gradually* occluded over 4 days, the dog's heart develops extensive collateral vessels that prevent myocardial infarction. After 4 days, the collateral vessels have done their job. The dog is now protected from heart attack. In spite of a completely occluded coronary artery, the dog will suffer no cardiac damage. Dr. Schaper states:

> *When the time to complete occlusion was 4 days, myocardial infarction was prevented due to growth-transformation of pre-existing collaterals. (46)*

The formation of well-developed collaterals has a survival benefit" protecting us from heart attack, serving as our own personal bypass operation, courtesy of mother nature. Dr. van der Hoeven, writing in *Heart* in 2013 says:

> *The use of Beta blockers is associated with well-developed collaterals, shedding new light on the potential action mode of this drug in patients with CAD. (47)*

This explains the value of medical treatment with OMT, optimal medical treatment with beta blockers and other cardiac drugs that buy time for our heart to develop collateral circulation.

Chest Pain Stimulates Collateral Vessels

If you are experiencing angina symptoms with typical chest pain, you might find comfort in knowing the angina actually stimulates growth of collateral circulation. Dr. Fujita writes in *Heart, in* 1987:

> *It is concluded that myocardial ischaemia (i.e., angina) is important in promoting collateral development in man as well as in laboratory animals. (70)*

EECP: Extracorporeal Counterpulsation

Formation of collateral vessels is one of the expected outcomes of a procedure called EECP, EKG-Gated Extracorporeal Counterpulsation. Thomas Cowan is a passionate advocate of EECP, which in his opinion makes angioplasty unnecessary. EECP is discussed in chapter 24.

Autonomic Nervous System-Parasympathetic vs Sympathetic

Dr. Cowan tells us something we already know. The heart is very sensitive to our emotional state. Our language is filled with idioms and phases relating to the heart, such as "*She broke my heart.*" People have been known to succumb from heart attack on the basis of a sudden severe emotional shock, fear, grief, etc. This is called the Broken Heart Syndrome, as described by Dr. Wittstein in the 2007 *Cleveland Clinic Journal of Medicine.* (48)

Our physiology colleagues have studied the nerves innervating the heart. (49,50) Lucky for us, the heartbeat is automatic, controlled by the autonomic nervous system consisting of the sympathetic branch that speeds up the heart rate and the parasympathetic branch (from the vagus nerve), which slows down the heart rate. (49–51)

Studies of the autonomic nervous system by monitoring heart rate variability (HRV) show that patients with reduced parasympathetic activity have higher risk for heart attack, especially after a prior myocardial infarction. (52) Dr. Juan Sztajzel says (2004):

> *Decreased HRV has been shown to be a strong predictor of increased cardiac and/or arrhythmic mortality, particularly in the post-MI setting. (52)*

Dr. Knut Sroka, an expert on the autonomic nervous system, reports that heart-attack victims will show a peculiar sudden drop-off of parasympathetic activity just prior to their heart attack. (53) This reduction in parasympathetic activity can be prevented by ouabain, an endogenous cardiac steroid that restores parasympathetic activity by enhancing release of its principal neurotransmitter ACH (acetylcholine). (54,55)

Dr. Sroka's 2004 article in *Zeitshrift for Cardiology* proposes that ischemic cardiac events can be triggered by the autonomic nervous system. This could certainly explain the reported cases of heart attacks with completely normal coronary arteries. Dr. Sroka says:

> *About three quarters of myocardial ischemic events are triggered by the autonomic nervous system. . . . (with) almost complete withdrawal of tonic vagal activity with increased sympathetic activity. (56)*

Vagal nerve activation has been suggested as a promising new treatment for prevention of cardiovascular disease. (57)

Preventing Heart Attacks with Ouabain-Medical Armamentarium

As mentioned in a previous chapter, cardiac drugs such as beta blockers, calcium-channel blockers, nitrates, aspirin, and other blood thinners are typically used for OMT of the stable angina patient. (58)

Enter the Cardiac Glycoside: Ouabain

Dr. Thomas Cowen differs from mainstream cardiology in his drug of choice for medical treatment of the stable angina patient. Dr. Cowan reports success using ouabain, a cardiac drug with a chemical structure similar to digitalis, which is derived from the foxglove plant. Ouabain is an old botanical called strophanthus (strodival), obtained from an African plant, and still in use by cardiologists in Germany, obtainable from local German pharmacies. Dr. Cowan reports that in his office practice this medication has been successful in preventing heart attacks.

In 1991, researchers discovered that ouabain from the strophanthus plant is identical to our own endogenous cardiac glycosides made by the adrenal gland. (2) Digoxin (digitalis from the foxglove plant) is another one of the endogenous cardiac glycosides.

Benefits in Cardiac Ischemia, Angina, and Infarction

Use of ouabain in both animal and human studies show striking benefits for prevention of myocardial ischemia and heart attack. (60–61) The ouabain preparation is also called strodival/strophanthum. (5–18).

Ouabain for Prevention and Treatment of Heart Attack

In 2010, Dr. Fürstenwerth wrote that Ouabain is the "*insulin of the heart*," because it modulates cardiac metabolism, and described intravenous ouabain (strophanthin) as the safest treatment for angina pectoris, including heart attack. (62) Dr. Fürstenwerth says:

> *The main benefit (of ouabain) is in prevention and treatment of acute heart attacks. (62)*

Summary

The story is familiar. A natural plant botanical substance, ouabain, sharing its identity with an endogenous hormone produced by the adrenal gland, exhibits striking health benefits for angina, ischemia, and prevention of heart attack. (62) Yet, this natural drug is largely ignored by mainstream cardiology because it cannot be patented, and therefore large controlled studies are lacking. I would strongly urge NIH funding of future studies on the use of ouabain for prevention of myocardial ischemia.

◆　◆　◆　◆　◆

♦ References for Chapter 18

1) Cowan, Thomas. "What Causes Heart Attacks ?," Townsend Letter May, 2014.

2) Schoner, Wilhelm, and Georgios Scheiner-Bobis. "Endogenous and exogenous cardiac glycosides and their mechanisms of action." American journal of cardiovascular drugs 7.3 (2007): 173–189.3)

4) "Human Heart, Cosmic Heart: A Doctor's Quest to Understand, Treat, and Prevent Cardiovascular Disease," by Thomas Cowan MD (2016) Chelsea Green Publishing Company.

5) Cardiac Infarction g-Strophanthin (Ouabain) – the Endogenous Hormone. Dr. Rainer Moser Diploma chemist

6) Rolf-Jurgen Petry, January 25, 2009, Strophanthin, ouabain available in German pharmacies

7) Dr. Debusmann What is Strophanthin? Dr. Wieland Debusmann

8) Ouabain the wasted opportunity by Knut Sroka, MD

9) deleted

10) Acidity Theory of Atherosclerosis – New Evidences," by Carlos E. T. B. Monteiro 2012

11) Roberts, William C. "Coronary arteries in fatal acute myocardial infarction." Circulation 45.1 (1972): 215–230.

12) Murakami, Tatsuaki, et al. "Intracoronary aspiration thrombectomy for acute myocardial infarction." American Journal of Cardiology 82.7 (1998): 839–844.

13) O'Neill, William W. "Coronary thrombosis during acute myocardial infarction: Roberts was right!." American Journal of Cardiology 82 (1998): 896–897.

14) Spain, David M., and Victoria A. Bradess. "The Relationship of Coronary Thrombosis to Coronary Atherosclerosis and Ischemic Heart Disease:(A Necropsy Study Covering A Period of 25 Years)." The American Journal of the Medical Sciences 240.6 (1960): 69–78.

15) deleted

16) Burch, G. E., C. Y. Tsui, and J. M. Harb. "Ischemic cardiomyopathy." American heart journal 83.3 (1972): 340–350.

17) PERSPECTIVE CUNICAL PRACTICE – Ouabain – the insulin of the heart. Int J Clin Pract, November 2010, 64, 12, 1591–1594

18) deleted

19) Baroldi, Giorgio. "Acute coronary occlusion as a cause of myocardial infarct and sudden coronary heart death." American Journal of Cardiology 16.6 (1965): 859–880.

21) Roberts, William C. "Coronary thrombosis and fatal myocardial ischemia." Circulation 49.1 (1974): 1–3.

22) Silver, Malcolm D., Giorgio Baroldi, and Fabio Mariani. "The relationship between acute occlusive coronary thrombi and myocardial infarction studied in 100 consecutive patients. "Circulation 61.2 (1980): 219–227.

23) Laredo, J. A. M. E. S., BRUCE P. Hamilton, and JOHN M. Hamlyn. "Ouabain is secreted by bovine adrenocortical cells." Endocrinology 135.2 (1994): 794–797.

24) Doris, PETER A., et al. "Ouabain production by cultured adrenal cells." Endocrinology 137.2 (1996): 533–539.

25) Foster, Richard H., Hernan Prat, and Ilan Rothman. "Is ouabain produced by the adrenal gland?." General Pharmacology: The Vascular System 31.4 (1998): 499–501.

26) Eliot, R. S., G. Baroldi, and A. Leone. "Necropsy studies in myocardial infarction with minimal or no coronary luminal reduction due to atherosclerosis." Circulation 49.6 (1974): 1127–1131.

27) Rosenblatt, Andrew, and A. R. T. H. U. R. Selzer. "The nature and clinical features of myocardial infarction with normal coronary arteriogram." Circulation 55.4 (1977): 578–580.

28) Betriu, Amadeo, et al. "Myocardial infarction with normal coronary arteries: a prospective clinical-angiographic study." American Journal of Cardiology 48.1 (1981): 28–32.

29) Salem, Bakr I., et al. "Acute Myocardial Infarction with "Normal" Coronary Arteries: Clinical, Angiographic Profiles with Ergonovine Testing." Texas Heart Institute Journal 12.1 (1985): 1.

30) Da Costa, A., et al. "Clinical characteristics, aetiological factors and long-term prognosis of myocardial infarction with an absolutely normal coronary angiogram; a 3-year follow-up study of 91 patients." European heart journal 22.16 (2001): 1459–1465.

31) Opherk, D., et al. "Coronary and left ventricular function in patients with normal coronarogram after clinically diagnosed infarct." Verhandlungen der Deutschen Gesellschaft fur Innere Medizin 84 (1978): 711.

32) Meierhenrich, R., et al. "Acute myocardial infarction in patients with angiographically normal coronary arteries: clinical features and medium-term follow-up." Zeitschrift fur Kardiologie 89.1 (2000): 36–42.

33) Sedlis, Steven P., et al. "Effect of PCI on long-term survival in patients with stable ischemic heart disease." New England Journal of Medicine 373.20 (2015): 1937–1946.

34) Boden, William E., et al. "Optimal medical therapy with or without PCI for stable coronary disease." New England Journal of Medicine 356.15 (2007): 1503–1516.

35) Schulman-Marcus, Joshua, et al. "Coronary revascularization vs. medical therapy following coronary-computed tomographic angiography in patients with low-, intermediate-and high-risk coronary artery disease: results from the CONFIRM long-term registry." European Heart Journal-Cardiovascular Imaging (2017): jew287.

36) Rihal, Charanjit S., et al. "Indications for coronary artery bypass surgery and percutaneous coronary intervention in chronic stable angina." Circulation 108.20 (2003): 2439–2445. Mayo Clinic 2003

37) Cohen, M. A. R. C., and K. PETER Rentrop. "Limitation of myocardial ischemia by collateral circulation during sudden controlled coronary artery occlusion in human subjects: a prospective study." Circulation 74.3 (1986): 469–476.

38) Meier, Pascal, et al. "The collateral circulation of the heart." BMC medicine 11.1 (2013): 143.

39) Gloekler, Steffen, et al. "Coronary collateral growth by external counterpulsation: a randomised controlled trial." Heart 96.3 (2010): 202–207.

40) Roth, D. M., et al. "Development of coronary collateral circulation in left circumflex Ameroid-occluded swine myocardium." American Journal of Physiology-Heart and Circulatory Physiology 253.5 (1987): H1279-H1288.

41) Chandrasekaran, B., and A. S. Kurbaan. "Myocardial infarction with angiographically normal coronary arteries." Journal of the Royal Society of Medicine 95.8 (2002): 398–400.

42) Joseph, Abraham, et al. "Manifestations of coronary atherosclerosis in young trauma victims—an autopsy study." Journal of the American College of Cardiology 22.2 (1993): 459–467.

43) Arbustini, Eloisa, et al. "Coronary thrombosis in non-cardiac death." Coronary artery disease 4.9 (1993): 751–759.

44) Hueb, Whady, et al. "Five-year follow-up of the Medicine, Angioplasty, or Surgery Study (MASS II): a randomized controlled clinical trial of 3 therapeutic strategies for multivessel coronary artery disease." Circulation 115.9 (2007): 1082–1089.

45) Holmes Jr, David R., and Malcolm R. Bell. "Left anterior descending artery stenosis: the widow maker revisited." Mayo Clinic Proceedings. Vol. 75. No. 11. Elsevier, 2000.

46) Schaper, W., and St Pasyk. "Influence of collateral flow on the ischemic tolerance of the heart following acute and subacute coronary occlusion." Circulation 53.3 Suppl (1976): I57–62.

47) van der Hoeven, Nina W., et al. "Clinical parameters associated with collateral development in patients with chronic total coronary occlusion." Heart 99.15 (2013): 1100–1105.

48) Wittstein, Ilan S. "The broken heart syndrome." Cleveland Clinic journal of medicine 74 (2007): S17.

49) Johnson, Christopher D., Sean Roe, and Etain A. Tansey. "Investigating autonomic control of the cardiovascular system: a battery of simple tests." Advances in physiology education 37.4 (2013): 401–404.

50) Klabunde, R. E. "Autonomic innervation of the heart and vasculature." (2008).

51) Hasan, Wohaib. "Autonomic cardiac innervation: development and adult plasticity." Organogenesis 9.3 (2013): 176–193.

52) Sztajzel, Juan. "Heart rate variability: a noninvasive electrocardiographic method to measure the autonomic nervous system." Swiss medical weekly 134.35–36 (2004): 514–522.

53) McAreavey, D., et al. "Cardiac parasympathetic activity during the early hours of acute myocardial infarction." Heart 62.3 (1989): 165–170.

54) Release of Acetylcholine from Synaptosomes." Journal of neurochemistry 58.3 (1992): 1038–1044.

55) Vyas, S., and R. M. Marchbanks. "The effect of ouabain on the release of [14C] acetylcholine and other substances from synaptosomes." Journal of neurochemistry 37.6 (1981): 1467–1474.

56) Sroka, Knut. "On the genesis of myocardial ischemia." Zeitschrift für Kardiologie 93.10 (2004): 768–783.

57) Zhao, Mei, et al. "Vagal nerve modulation: a promising new therapeutic approach for cardiovascular diseases." Clinical and Experimental Pharmacology and Physiology 39.8 (2012): 701–705.

58) Shavelle, David M. "Long term medical treatment of stable coronary disease." HEART-LONDON-BMJ PUBLISHING GROUP 93.11 (2007): 1473.

59) deleted

60) Vatner, STEPHEN F., and Hank Baig. "Comparison of the effects of ouabain and isoproterenol on ischemic myocardium of conscious dogs." Circulation 58.4 (1978): 654–662.

61) Sharma, B., et al. "Clinical, electrocardiographic, and haemodynamic effects of digitalis (ouabain) in angina pectoris." British Heart Journal 34.6 (1972): 631.

62) Fürstenwerth, Hauke. "Ouabain–the insulin of the heart." International journal of clinical practice 64.12 (2010): 1591–1594.

63) deleted

64) Cardiac Glycosides. by Arthur Stoll, Published by Pharmaceutical Press, (1937)., London

65) Schmermund, Axel, et al. "Coronary atherosclerosis in unheralded sudden coronary death under age 50: histo-pathologic comparison with 'healthy' subjects dying out of hospital." Atherosclerosis 155.2 (2001): 499–508.

66) Hillebrand, Stefanie, et al. "Heart rate variability and first cardiovascular event in populations without known cardiovascular disease: meta-analysis and dose–response meta-regression." Europace 15.5 (2013): 742–749.

67) Liao, Duanping, et al. "Cardiac autonomic function and incident coronary heart disease: a population-based case-cohort study: the ARIC Study." American Journal of Epidemiology 145.8 (1997): 696–706.

68) McAreavey, D., et al. "Cardiac parasympathetic activity during the early hours of acute myocardial infarction." Heart 62.3 (1989): 165–170.

69) Seiler, Christian. "The human coronary collateral circulation." Heart 89.11 (2003): 1352–1357.

70) Fujita, M., et al. "Importance of angina for development of collateral circulation." Heart 57.2 (1987): 139–143.

71) Yoshida, Michi, et al. "Effect of collateral circulation on myocardial protection in patients with acute myocardial infarction: comparison of technetium-99m-tetrofosmin myocardial single photon emission computed tomography and coronary angiography." Journal of cardiology 47.3 (2006): 115–121.

72) Schoner, Wilhelm, and Georgios Scheiner-Bobis. "Endogenous and exogenous cardiac glycosides: their roles in hypertension, salt metabolism, and cell growth." American Journal of Physiology-Cell Physiology 293.2 (2007): C509-C536.

73) Schoner, Wilhelm, and Georgios Scheiner-Bobis. "Endogenous cardiac glycosides: hormones using the sodium pump as signal transducer." Seminars in nephrology. Vol. 25. No. 5. Elsevier, 2005.

The "Flip-Flop" on Estrogen and Heart Disease

MEDICAL SCIENCE HAS DONE A flip-flop on estrogen and coronary heart disease. Before 2002, forty observational studies proved that estrogen prevents heart disease in women. Three medical societies published guidelines offering hormone replacement for women, and it was considered unethical medical malpractice to do otherwise. It was believed that estrogen in young females conferred protection from coronary artery disease, and estrogen replacement prevented coronary artery disease in postmenopausal women.

2002 WHI Study with Premarin and Medroxyprogesterone (Prempro)

The tables were turned in 2002 when the Women's Health Initiative (WHI) was terminated early because of increased heart disease in the Prempro-treated group. (17) The failure of the WHI randomized controlled trial to show cardiac benefit for the Prempro group arrived in the wake of a number of RCT studies in the 1990s, such as the HERS trial, all expecting the same cardio-protection shown in observational and animal studies. Yet, the result was quite the opposite: All these RCTs failed to show reduction in heart disease for estrogen hormone users. (22) The question is, *"Why did these studies fail? "*

The Wrong Hormones and the Wrong Age Group

The WHI First-Arm, the HERS study, and other RCTs (randomized controlled trials) in the 1990s used the wrong hormones. They used a synthetic "progestin" called medroxyprogesterone. They also used the wrong age group, women who were past their 60s, fifteen years out from the menopausal transition.

Dr. Barrett-Conner 2003: Estrogen is a Failure!

In 2003, Dr. Elizabeth Barrett-Conner lamented the failure of estrogen to prevent coronary heart disease (CHD) in postmenopausal women:

> *The failure to find cardioprotective effects in any of the several clinical trials with CHD outcomes offers little hope that postmenopausal HT (Hormone Replacement) will prevent heart disease. The results, unexpected and unwelcome, are nonetheless definitive and are likely to extend beyond the studied treatment regimens. (1)*

Of course, the above dramatic comment by Dr. Barrett-Conner is completely wrong, as you will see below.

2011 – A Massive Flip-Flop, Estrogen Is Indeed Cardio-Protective

The 2011 *JAMA* report of the 11-year follow-up of the Second Arm (Premarin-only) of the Women's Health Initiative (WHI), clearly showed that estrogen reduces mortality from heart disease. Estrogen not only reduces heart attacks, estrogen also reduces all-cause mortality. (15,16)

However, protection was conferred only on the 50-to-60-year age group, and not on the older women, who had already experienced 10 to 20 years of hormone deficiency. In addition, this protection was lost or reduced when a synthetic progestin, medroxyprogesterone, was added to the hormone cocktail.

The data from the 11-year follow-up of the Second Arm of the WHI shows a number of important findings. The Second Arm study included women after hysterectomy using Premarin alone. (15)

For the "younger" age group (age 50–60 years), HRT with Premarin alone provided an astounding 41% reduction in coronary artery disease, 46% reduction in myocardial infarctions, and 27% reduction in all-cause mortality. (15) In addition, there was a 20–30% reduction in breast cancer. When one puts all the age groups together, the benefit is NULL. However, when one looks at the 50–60 age group, the benefits of starting hormone replacement immediately after the hormone decline of menopause are striking.

Estrogen is effective in preventing atherosclerotic coronary artery disease in the 50–60-year age group if started right away at the initiation of menopause. Estrogen alone is ineffective for preventing coronary artery disease when introduced 10 or 20 years after menopause.

Twenty-Three RCTs Re-Examined: Behold a Benefit for Younger Post-Menopause

Moreover, when one goes back to the RCTs done in the 1990s that failed to show a cardiovascular benefit for estrogen and re-examines the data set for the younger postmenopausal age group, there is a 30–40% reduction in cardiovascular disease risk. (21) This was confirmed in a 2006 meta-analysis of 23 RCTs of hormone replacement by Dr. Salpeter, revealing the same 30–40% decrease in CV risk in young postmenopausal women. (21)

Don't Wait

The take-home message for women entering menopause is: *"Don't Wait"* to start bio-identical hormone replacement immediately upon onset of menopausal symptoms.

Hormonal decline of menopause is a health risk leading to onset of chronic inflammation, chronic degenerative disease, osteoarthritis, osteoporosis, cognitive impairment, and cognitive dysfunction, as well as coronary atherosclerosis.

Two Coronary Calcium Score Studies Are
Consistent with Cardio-Protection

Coronary artery calcium score has emerged over the last decade as a highly accurate surrogate marker for coronary artery plaque and heart-disease risk. Two coronary calcium score studies evaluated in women from the WHI study group showed striking benefits for the Premarin-alone users, but not for the Premarin-Progestin combination users.

Dr. JoAnn Manson's study measured calcium score at the end of the 8.7-year observation period for "younger" women in the 50–59 age group. (18) The women using Premarin alone had a 60% lower calcium score compared to placebo users. Dr. JoAnn Manson writes in the *New England Journal of Medicine* (2005):

> *These findings, in conjunction with the suggestion of a reduced risk of clinical coronary events among women treated with conjugated equine estrogens (Premarin) in this age group, are consistent with previous evidence from laboratory, animal, and observational studies. (18)*

A second study was published in 2005 in the *Journal of Women's Health* by Dr. Budoff. This study performed two consecutive calcium scores one year apart, examining the progression of the calcium score. For the Premarin-alone treated women, the study showed an increase of only 9%, compared to 22% for non-users. The Premarin-alone users had a 63% reduction in progression of calcification compared to non-users. Premarin-Progestin combination users had a 24% annual increase, about the same as non-users (19). A 2007 study in the *American Journal of Cardiology* by Dr. Becker in Germany showed the same findings, i.e., that the Premarin-Progestin combination failed to reduce progression of calcium score compared to non-hormone users.

How Does Estrogen Prevent Coronary Artery Disease ?

An excellent 2009 article by Dr. Bechlioulis reviews the benefits of estrogen in preventing endothelial dysfunction, the initiating step in atherosclerosis. (20) Flow-mediated dilatation (FMD) of the brachial artery is a handy tool for evaluating endothelial dysfunction. Studies using FMD show that estrogen deficiency is linked to endothelial dysfunction in postmenopausal women, women with premature menopause, surgically induced menopause, and other groups with low estrogen levels. (20)

Estrogen is Anti-Inflammatory: Basic Science Studies

A number of basic science studies in animals and humans show that estrogen has a profound anti-inflammatory effect, and this explains much of the cardio-protection. (23–28, 31)

Carotid Plaque Study from Italy: Less Inflammation in the Plaque

An elegant study from Italy examined inflammatory markers and cells in actual carotid artery plaques surgically removed from women using hormone replacement and compared them to a control group of women who were not using hormone replacement. (30) In women using hormone replacement, the authors found considerable reduction of inflammatory cells and markers in the plaque material. (30)

Estrogen Upregulates EPCs

The endothelial progenitor cell (EPC) has been recognized as an important component of cardio-protection, and estrogen upregulates the EPCs, conferring protection in the mouse model of myocardial infarction. The administration of estrogen stimulates faster recovery after ischemic injury by increasing EPCs and neo-angiogeneisis (29)

Estradiol Metabolite Prevents Atherosclerosis

Dr. Johan Bourghardt reported in *Endocrinology* (2007) that a metabolite of estradiol called 2-methoxyestradiol reduces atherosclerotic lesion formation in female apolipoprotein E-deficient mice. (32) The author commented:

The anti-atherogenic activity of an estradiol metabolite lacking estrogen receptor activating capacity may argue that trials on cardiovascular effects of hormone replacement therapy should use estradiol rather than other estrogens. (32)

Drs. Howard Hodis and Wendy Mack Sum It Up (8,9,10)

The cardio-protection of estrogen is best described by Drs. Howard Hodis and Wendy Mack in a series of articles from 2008 to 2011. The authors state that for women in the 50–60 year age group, in the immediate postmenopausal period, all of the randomized controlled trials are in agreement with the observational and animal studies. These clearly show a cardio-protective effect for postmenopausal estrogen replacement with a 40–50% reduction in "cardiac events." (8,9,10).

Drs. Hodis and Mack point out that results for this age group are similar to all the preceding observational (1) and animal studies (8-9). This is called the "window of opportunity" for hormonal replacement in the 40–50 age window. Estrogen (Premarin) is successful in reducing heart disease risk for the 50–60 age group, and ineffective for the over-60 age group. (15,16)

This makes sense when considering that hormonal decline of natural or surgically induced menopause is associated with degenerative diseases such as coronary artery disease, osteoporosis, osteoarthritis, and cognitive decline, all of which are associated with increased mortality rate (11,12) (26) (34).

Avoid Synthetic Monster Hormones

In addition, it is now clear that women must avoid synthetic hormones, such as medroxyprogesterone, a "progestin" called Provera. This synthetic monster hormone causes heart disease and opposes the cardio-protective effects of Estrogen. (19) It was also found to increase breast cancer risk in numerous studies. It is now clear that ovarian hormones, estradiol and progesterone, are the preferred hormone choice. These ovarian hormones are bio-identical.

Avoid Blood Clots with Transdermal Estrogen

A 2010 report by Dr. Leonard Speroff in *Climacteric* points out that topical estrogen is preferred over pill forms (such as Premarin). The transdermal route is not associated with increased blood clots, since it avoids having to first pass through the liver. (14) This has been confirmed by others.

Statin Anti-Cholesterol Drug to Prevent Heart Disease in Women?

Cholesterol studies with statin drugs show no health benefit for women, yet many postmenopausal women come to my office on statin drugs prescribed by their primary care doctor or cardiologist to reduce cholesterol. These women are obsessed with their cholesterol level. They are all worried their cholesterol is too high. They are all "terrorized" by the drug-marketing television campaigns. The cardiologists and primary doctors go along with the ruse and hand out statin drugs to women quite freely. Statin drugs come with horrendous adverse side effects that I see every day in my office. To give such a drug treatment without any known benefit to outweigh the adverse effect is a form of mistreatment and abuse that must be halted.

Adverse Effects of Statin Drugs

Adverse effects of statin drugs are nicely summarized in a 2008 article by Beatrice Golomb, MD, in the *American Journal of Cardiovascular Drugs*. Statin drugs are mitochondrial toxins that deplete co-enzyme Q10 levels, causing neuropathy, myopathy, congestive heart failure, transient global amnesia, erectile dysfunction, dementia, blood-sugar elevation, and other disorders. (50)

No Benefit for Women with Statin Drugs

The reality is that statin drugs do not reduce mortality from heart disease in women, nor do they reduce all-cause mortality. This data is summarized in articles by Dr. Judith Walsh in JAMA (2004), Dr. Petretta (2010) in the International Journal of Cardiology, and Dr. Ray 2010 in the Archives of Internal Medicine (38-40).

Lipid-lowering with statin drugs is ill-advised, according to Drs. Hodis and Mack:

Lipid-lowering therapy, predominantly with HMG-CoA reductase inhibitors [statin drugs] is the mainstay for the primary prevention of

CHD in women. The cumulated data however, do not provide convincing evidence for the significant reduction of CHD with lipid-lowering therapy relative to placebo when used for primary prevention of CHD in women and there is no evidence that such therapy reduces overall mortality.(8)

Observations Suggesting Estrogen Is Cardio-Protective for Women (1):

- Heart disease is uncommon in women before the age of menopause.
- Heart disease is more common in women who have a premature natural menopause.
- Heart disease is more common in young women who have had both ovaries removed.
- Heart disease is less common in women who take HT after menopause.

The Short History of Women's Hormone Replacement and Heart Disease

1920–1939: Estradiol synthesized (1938)

1940–1949:: Premarin introduced (1942)

1983–1987: Observational Studies on RT and Heart Disease. The first observational studies of the benefits of RT (hormone replacement) were published by Trudy Bush in 1983 and 1987 showing reduction in cardiovascular disease and total mortality in hormone users. (2,3)

1991: 50% Reduction in Mortality from Heart Disease—11 studies. Dr. Conner reported that 11 studies showed a 50% reduction in mortality from heart disease for post-menopausal women using estrogen alone (without a progestin). (4) She writes: *"Most, but not all, studies of hormone replacement therapy in post-menopausal women show around a 50% reduction in risk of a coronary event in women using unopposed oral estrogen."* (4)

1992: Dr. Deborah Grady publishes a landmark meta-analysis in the Annals of Internal Medicine, reviewing the medical literature since 1970 showing postmenopausal estrogen replacement reduces risk of heart disease in women and reduces fracture risk as well. (5)

1992: Three Medical Organizations Endorse Estrogen Therapy to Prevent Heart Disease. Also in 1992, three medical organizations, the American College of Physicians, the American College of Obstetrics and Gynecology and the American Heart Association proposed guidelines that all postmenopausal women should be offered estrogen hormone replacement to prevent heart disease. (5,6,7)

1995–1999: Prempro, the first combination Hormone Replacement pill is introduced, and a HERS study (1998) using Prempro reports early increased heart disease risk.

2002–2003: WHI (First Arm, using Prempro) reports increased heart disease, stroke, and breast cancer, WHI continues unopposed estrogen arm (Premarin alone Second Arm), FDA requires black box warning for all post-menopausal estrogens with or without progestin.

2003: Dr. Barrett-Conner wrote an article in JCEM summarizing the previous three decades of research on estrogen and heart disease. She observes:

Women have a lower risk of heart disease than men of comparable age, with roughly twice the mortality for males compared to females. (1)

2004 : WHI Second Arm published showing less breast cancer and less heart disease in hormone users (Premarin only) (15)

2011: WHI Second Arm 11-year follow-up data published showing coronary artery disease reduced by half in "younger" 50–60-year-old women using Premarin alone without a progestin. (15,16)

Conclusion

Don't wait. The cardio-protective benefits of estrogen replacement are greatest at the initiation of menopause, and health benefits diminish after the many years in which degenerative disease is allowed to progress. Do not wait to start Hormone Replacement. The health benefits are greatest when starting hormone replacement at the initiation of menopause. Dr. Schierbeck writing in 2012 in BMJ says:

After 10 years of randomized treatment, women receiving hormone replacement therapy early after menopause had a significantly reduced risk of mortality, heart failure, or myocardial infarction, without any apparent increase in risk of cancer, venous thromboembolism, or stroke. (42)

The obvious conclusion is that for postmenopausal women, bio-identical hormones are much more effective than statin drugs in reducing risk of a "cardiac event." Women should stop statin drugs and instead switch to bio-identical hormone replacement for cardio-protection.

◆　◆　◆　◆　◆

◆ References for Chapter 19

1) Barrett-Connor, Elizabeth. "An epidemiologist looks at hormones and heart disease in women." The Journal of Clinical Endocrinology & Metabolism 88.9 (2003): 4031–4042.

2) Bush, Trudy L., et al. "Estrogen use and all-cause mortality." Jama 249.7 (1983): 903–906.

3) Bush, Trudy L., et al. "Cardiovascular mortality and noncontraceptive use of estrogen in women: results from the Lipid Research Clinics Program Follow-up Study." Circulation 75.6 (1987): 1102–1109.

4) Barrett-Connor, Elizabeth, and Trudy L. Bush. "Estrogen and coronary heart disease in women." Jama 265.14 (1991): 1861–1867.

5) Grady, Deborah, et al. "Hormone therapy to prevent disease and prolong life in postmenopausal women." Annals of internal medicine 117.12 (1992): 1016–1037.

6) Grady, Deborah, et al. "GUIDELINES FOR COUNSELING POSTMENOPAUSAL WOMEN ABOUT PREVENTIVE HORMONE-THERAPY." Annals of internal medicine 117.12 (1992): 1038–1041.

7) Andrews, William C., et al. "Guidelines for counseling women on the management of menopause." Washington, DC: Jacobs Institute of Women's Health Expert Panel on Menopause Counseling (2000).

8) Hodis, Howard N., and Wendy J. Mack. "A "window of opportunity:" the reduction of coronary heart disease and total mortality with menopausal therapies is age- and time-dependent." Brain research 1379 (2011): 244–252.

9) Hodis, Howard N., and Wendy J. Mack. "Postmenopausal hormone therapy and cardiovascular disease in perspective." Clinical obstetrics and gynecology 51.3 (2008): 564.

10) Utian, Wulf H. "In Perspective: Estrogen Therapy Safely and Effectively Reduces Total Mortality and Coronary Heart Disease in Recently Menopausal Women."

11) Lubiszewska, Barbara, et al. "The impact of early menopause on risk of coronary artery disease (PREmature Coronary Artery Disease In Women–PRECADIW case-control study)." European journal of preventive cardiology 19.1 (2012): 95–101.

12) Maclaran, Kate, Etienne Horner, and Nick Panay. "Premature ovarian failure: long-term sequelae." Menopause International 16.1 (2010): 38–41.

13) Clarkson, Thomas B. "Estrogen effects on arteries vary with stage of reproductive life and extent of subclinical atherosclerosis progression." Menopause 14.3 (2007): 373–384

13a)Williams, J. Koudy, and Irma Suparto. "Hormone replacement therapy and cardiovascular disease: lessons from a monkey model of postmenopausal women." ILAR journal 45.2 (2004): 139–146.

13b)Adams, Michael R., et al. "Medroxyprogesterone acetate antagonizes inhibitory effects of conjugated equine estrogens on coronary artery atherosclerosis." Arteriosclerosis, thrombosis, and vascular biology 17.1 (1997): 217–221.

14) Speroff, L. "Transdermal hormone therapy and the risk of stroke and venous thrombosis." Climacteric 13.5 (2010): 429–432.

15) LaCroix, Andrea Z., et al. "Health outcomes after stopping conjugated equine estrogens among postmenopausal women with prior hysterectomy: a randomized controlled trial." Jama 305.13 (2011): 1305–1314.

16) Anderson, Garnet L., et al. "Conjugated equine oestrogen and breast cancer incidence and mortality in postmenopausal women with hysterectomy: extended follow-up of the Women's Health Initiative randomised placebo-controlled trial." The lancet oncology 13.5 (2012): 476–486.

17) Writing Group for the Women's Health Initiative Investigators. "Risks and benefits of estrogen plus progestin in healthy postmenopausal women: principal results from the Women's Health Initiative randomized controlled trial." Jama 288.3 (2002): 321–333.

18) Manson, JoAnn E., et al. "Estrogen therapy and coronary-artery calcification." New England Journal of Medicine 356.25 (2007): 2591–2602.

19) Budoff, Matthew J., et al. "Effects of hormone replacement on progression of coronary calcium as measured by electron beam tomography." Journal of women's health 14.5 (2005): 410–417.

19) Weinberg, Nicole, et al. "Physical activity, hormone replacement therapy, and the presence of coronary calcium in midlife women." Women & health 52.5 (2012): 423–436.

20) Bechlioulis, A. R. I. S., et al. "Menopause and hormone therapy: from vascular endothelial function to cardiovascular disease." Hellenic J Cardiol 50.4 (2009): 303–15.

21) Salpeter, Shelley R., et al. "Brief report: coronary heart disease events associated with hormone therapy in younger and older women." Journal of general internal medicine 21.4 (2006): 363–366.

22) Grady, Deborah, et al. "Cardiovascular disease outcomes during 6.8 years of hormone therapy: Heart and Estrogen/progestin Replacement Study follow-up (HERS II)." Jama 288.1 (2002): 49–57.

23) Miller, Virginia M., and Sue P. Duckles. "Vascular actions of estrogens: functional implications." Pharmacological reviews 60.2 (2008): 210–241.

24) Xing, Dongqi, et al. "Estrogen and mechanisms of vascular protection." Arteriosclerosis, thrombosis, and vascular biology 29.3 (2009): 289–295.

25) Yang, Xiao-Ping, and Jane F. Reckelhoff. "Estrogen, hormonal replacement therapy and cardiovascular disease." Current opinion in nephrology and hypertension 20.2 (2011): 133.

26) Parker, William H., et al. "Ovarian conservation at the time of hysterectomy and long-term health outcomes in the nurses' health study." Obstetrics and gynecology 113.5 (2009): 1027.

27) Miller, Andrew P., et al. "Hormone replacement therapy and inflammation: interactions in cardiovascular disease." Hypertension 42.4 (2003): 657–663.

28) Mendelsohn, Michael E., and Richard H. Karas. "The protective effects of estrogen on the cardiovascular system." New England journal of medicine 340.23 (1999): 1801–1811.

29) Hamada, Hiromichi, et al. "Estrogen receptors α and β mediate contribution of bone marrow–derived endothelial progenitor cells to functional recovery after myocardial infarction." Circulation 114.21 (2006): 2261–2270.

30) Marfella, Raffaele, et al. "Proteasome Activity as a Target of Hormone Replacement Therapy–Dependent Plaque Stabilization in Postmenopausal Women." Hypertension 51.4 (2008): 1135–1141.

31) Nofer, Jerzy-Roch. "Estrogens and atherosclerosis: insights from animal models and cell systems." Journal of molecular endocrinology 48.2 (2012): R13-R29.

32) Bourghardt, Johan, et al. "The endogenous estradiol metabolite 2-methoxyestradiol reduces atherosclerotic lesion formation in female apolipoprotein E-deficient mice." Endocrinology 148.9 (2007): 4128–4132.

33) Rocca, Walter A., et al. "Increased risk of cognitive impairment or dementia in women who underwent oophorectomy before menopause." Neurology 69.11 (2007): 1074–1083.

34) Rivera, Cathleen M., et al. "Increased cardiovascular mortality following early bilateral oophorectomy." Menopause (New York, NY) 16.1 (2009): 15.

35) Recker, Robert R., et al. "The effect of low-dose continuous estrogen and progesterone therapy with calcium and vitamin D on bone in elderly women: a randomized, controlled trial." Annals of internal medicine 130.11 (1999): 897–904.

36) Løkkegaard, E., et al. "The association between early menopause and risk of ischaemic heart disease: influence of hormone therapy." Maturitas 53.2 (2006): 226–233.

37) Howell, Anthony and Cuzick, Jack, "Oestrogen and breast cancer: results from the WHI trial" The Lancet Oncology, 7 March 2012

38) Walsh, Judith ME, and Michael Pignone. "Drug treatment of hyperlipidemia in women." Jama 291.18 (2004): 2243–2252.

39) Petretta, Mario, et al. "Impact of gender in primary prevention of coronary heart disease with statin therapy: a meta-analysis." International journal of cardiology 138.1 (2010): 25–31.

40) Ray, Kausik K., et al. "Statins and all-cause mortality in high-risk primary prevention: a meta-analysis of 11 randomized controlled trials involving 65 229 participants." Archives of internal medicine 170.12 (2010): 1024–1031.

41) Grodstein, Francine, et al. "A prospective, observational study of postmenopausal hormone therapy and primary prevention of cardiovascular disease." Annals of internal medicine 133.12 (2000): 933–941.

42) Schierbeck, Louise Lind, et al. "Effect of hormone replacement therapy on cardiovascular events in recently postmenopausal women: randomised trial." Bmj 345 (2012): e6409.43)

43) Miller, Virginia M., and Sue P. Duckles. "Vascular actions of estrogens: functional implications." Pharmacological reviews 60.2 (2008): 210–241.

44) Fournier, Agnès, Franco Berrino, and Françoise Clavel-Chapelon. "Unequal risks for breast cancer associated with different hormone replacement therapies: results from the E3N cohort study." Breast cancer research and treatment 107.1 (2008): 103–111.

45) Jordan, V. Craig, and Leslie G. Ford. "Paradoxical clinical effect of estrogen on breast cancer risk: a "new" biology of estrogen-induced apoptosis." Cancer prevention research 4.5 (2011): 633–637.

46) Brünner, N., et al. "Effect of 17 β-oestradiol on growth curves and flow cytometric DNA distribution of two human breast carcinomas grown in nude mice." British journal of cancer 47.5 (1983): 641..

47) LaCroix, Andrea Z., et al. "Health outcomes after stopping conjugated equine estrogens among postmenopausal women with prior hysterectomy: a randomized controlled trial." Jama 305.13 (2011): 1305–1314.

48) Jungheim, Emily S., and Graham A. Colditz. "Short-term use of unopposed estrogen: a balance of inferred risks and benefits." Jama 305.13 (2011): 1354–1355.

49) Anderson, Garnet L., et al. "Conjugated equine oestrogen and breast cancer incidence and mortality in postmenopausal women with hysterectomy: extended follow-up of the Women's Health Initiative randomised placebo-controlled trial." The lancet oncology 13.5 (2012): 476–486.

50) 50) Golomb, Beatrice A., and Marcella A. Evans. "Statin adverse effects." American Journal of Cardiovascular Drugs 8.6 (2008): 373-418.

51) Estrogen taken alone is linked to lower breast cancer risk By Shari Roan, Los Angeles Times March 7, 2012 LA Times.

52) Estrogen Protects Against Breast Cancer Long After Treatment By: MARY ANN MOON, Internal Medicine News Digital Network

53) Estrogen Lowers Breast Cancer and Heart Attack Risk in Some By TARA PARKER-POPE April 5, 2011, New York Times.

54) Estrogen pills reduce breast cancer risk in study of menopausal women By CBS News Staff

55) Writing Group for the Women's Health Initiative Investigators. "Effects of conjugated equine estrogen in postmenopausal women with hysterectomy: the Women's Health Initiative randomized controlled trial." JAMA 291 (2004): 1701–1712.

56) Chlebowski, Rowan T., et al. "Influence of estrogen plus progestin on breast cancer and mammography in healthy postmenopausal women: the Women's Health Initiative Randomized Trial." Jama 289.24 (2003): 3243–3253.

57) Hyde, Zoe, et al. "Low free testosterone predicts mortality from cardiovascular disease but not other causes: the Health in Men Study." The Journal of Clinical Endocrinology & Metabolism 97.1 (2012): 179–189.

58) Hyde, Zoe, et al. "Low free testosterone predicts mortality from cardiovascular disease but not other causes: the Health in Men Study." The Journal of Clinical Endocrinology & Metabolism 97.1 (2012): 179–189.

59) Khaw, Kay-Tee, et al. "Endogenous testosterone and mortality due to all causes, cardiovascular disease, and cancer in men: European prospective investigation into cancer in Norfolk (EPIC-Norfolk) Prospective Population Study." Circulation 116.23 (2007): 2694–2701.

60) Shores, Molly M., et al. "Low serum testosterone and mortality in male veterans." Archives of internal medicine 166.15 (2006): 1660–1665.

61) Laughlin, Gail A., Elizabeth Barrett-Connor, and Jaclyn Bergstrom. "Low serum testosterone and mortality in older men." The Journal of Clinical Endocrinology & Metabolism 93.1 (2008): 68–75.

62) Stevenson, John C. "The Effect of Menopause and HRT on Coronary Heart Disease." Pre-Menopause, Menopause and Beyond. Springer, Cham, 2018. 187–193.

<table>
<tr><td>CHAPTER
20</td><td>**Thyroid Hormone Prevents
Atherosclerotic Disease**</td></tr>
</table>

IN 1976, DR. BRODA BARNES reported that having a low thyroid is associated with heart attack. (1–5)   How did he discover the connection between low thyroid and heart disease? Barnes took summer vacations in Graz, Austria, every year to study autopsy files. Graz has a high prevalence of thyroid disorders, and anyone in Graz who died over the previous 100 years required an autopsy to determine cause of death, as mandated by the authorities. This rather large amount of autopsy data showed that low-thyroid patients survived the usual childhood infectious diseases thanks to the invention of antibiotics. However, years later, they were prone to develop heart disease. Barnes also found that thyroid treatment was protective in preventing heart attacks, based on his own clinical experience. Likewise, he found that adding thyroid medication was beneficial at preventing the onset of vascular disease in diabetics. New research like the Hunt Study confirms that Barnes was right all along, creating a paradigm shift in thyroid treatment. (19)

The Hunt Study: Thyroid Function and Heart Disease

TSH is thyroid stimulating hormone made by the pituitary gland. TSH actually stimulates the thyroid gland to make more thyroid hormone and can therefore be used as a barometer of thyroid function. If thyroid function is low, the pituitary makes more TSH to stimulate the thyroid gland, which in turn, makes more thyroid hormone. Mainstream medicine regards the TSH as the single most important test for determining thyroid function. High TSH means low thyroid function, and a low TSH means normal or high thyroid function.

What Did the Hunt Study Find?

The Hunt Study from the April 2008 *Archives of Internal Medicine* examined mortality from coronary heart disease (CHD) and TSH level. The authors conclude:

> *The results indicate that relatively low but clinically normal thyroid function may increase the risk of fatal CHD. (19)*

The study measured thyroid function with the TSH test in 17,000 women and 8,000 men with no known thyroid or heart disease. All patients had "normal" TSH levels, meaning the TSH values were in the lab reference range of 0.5 to 3.5. The women were stratified into three groups, lower TSH, intermediate, and upper TSH levels, and mortality from heart disease was recorded over an 8-year observation period.

Seventy Percent Increase in Heart Disease Mortality for TSH in Upper Normal Range

The Hunt study found that group with the higher TSH had a 70% increased mortality from heart disease compared to the lower TSH group. (19) Remember, all these TSH values were in the normal lab range. *This finding is earthshaking!* This suggests reducing TSH to the low end of "normal" by taking a thyroid hormone pill can effectively reduce death from cardiovascular disease by 70%. This mortality benefit is mind boggling and far exceeds any drug intervention available.

The above concept was confirmed in 2012 by Dr. Salman Razvi, who studied patients with subclinical hypothyroidism treated with levothyroxine over 7 years. The addition of thyroid medication provided a 57% reduction in cardiovascular events in the 50-to-70-year-old group. (5)

Thyroid and the Immune System

Recent studies reveal the close interrelation of the immune system and thyroid function, just as Broda Barnes proposed decades ago. The ability to battle and withstand an infectious insult was studied in hypothyroid mice in 2014 by Dr. Cristiana Perrotta from Milan, Italy. (11)

Dr. Perrotta studied a hypothyroid mouse model and found that T3 (tri-iodothyronine thyroid hormone) significantly protected mice against endotoxemia induced by intraperitoneal (into the body cavity) injections of lipopolysaccharide (LPS). (11)

Dr. Perrotta injected hypothyroid mice with gram-negative bacteria lipopolysaccharide to induce endotoxemia. The hypothyroid mice had 90% mortality after 96 hours. However, when the hypothyroid mice were injected with T3 (thyroid hormone) for 5 days before gram-negative endotoxemia, they were now protected from death with 70% survival. The T3- (thyroid-hormone-) treated mice enjoyed the greatest survival and best outcome. This is an impressive demonstration of the importance of thyroid hormone for boosting our immune system and protecting us from infectious disease.

Why is this important for heart disease prevention? Remember chapter 13, which was devoted to the LPS theory of heart disease? Thyroid hormone helps the immune system defend against LPS low-level endotoxemia, thus clearing the gram-negative organisms from the bloodstream and preventing seeding of the atherosclerotic plaque with polymicrobial biofilm.

Cholesterol Helps Clear LPS Low-Level Endotoxemia

Another defense against LPS and low-level endotoxemia is cholesterol itself. Cholesterol is part of our immune defense system. Both animal and human studies show cholesterol inactivates LPS and bacterial endotoxin, serving as a second line of defense against translocated LPS. (15–16) Dr. Sandek explains the ability of cholesterol to detoxify LPS as the "endotoxin-lipoprotein hypothesis." (17) Dr. D. Pajkrt studied this hypothesis in vivo with human volunteers, infusing reconstituted HDL cholesterol just prior to endotoxin infusion. The authors conclude:

> *The HDL cholesterol infusion . . . dramatically reduced the endotoxin-induced inflammatory response, reduced inflammatory cytokines, cell activation, and clinical symptoms in humans . . . partly caused by neutralization of endotoxin by reconstituted HDL cholesterol. (15)*

As one might expect, low HDL cholesterol level is a predictor of increased mortality in patients with endotoxemia from sepsis. (18) So, we must conclude that if the LPS theory of heart disease is correct, and atherosclerotic plaque is infected biofilm, then higher cholesterol levels, not lower, are beneficial in clearing the LPS from the bloodstream and defending against seeding of atherosclerotic plaque with micro-organisms. In this scenario, reducing cholesterol levels is misguided.

Statin Drugs or Thyroid to Prevent Heart Disease in Women?

Decades of published statin drug studies show that statin drugs simply don't work for women and don't reduce mortality from heart disease in women. On the other hand, the HUNT study shows that TSH levels in the lower normal range provide a 70% reduction in heart disease mortality for women. This can be accomplished safely with inexpensive thyroid medication under a physician's supervision. For women concerned about preventing heart disease, this is good news, pointing out a natural alternative to statin drugs that works better.

Natural Thyroid is Better

Rather than using T4 only medications such as Levothyroxine, natural desiccated thyroid is preferable. We have seen better clinical results with the natural thyroid preparations compared to the T4-only medications.

How to Design a Better Hunt Study

How would I design an even better Hunt Study? That's easy. Include another group of patients with TSH levels above and below the study group, namely, below 0.5, and above 3.5. I would also include data on annual CAT coronary calcium scores. I would predict that the lower TSH group (below 0.5) would have even less heart disease than the higher TSH group, and that coronary calcium score would go up as TSH went up.

◆ ◆ ◆ ◆ ◆

◆ References for Chapter 20

1) Barnes, Broda O. "Prophylaxis of ischaemic heart-disease by thyroid therapy." The Lancet 274.7095 (1959): 149–152.

2) Barnes, Broda Otto, and Charlotte W. Barnes. Solved: the riddle of heart attacks. Robinson Press, 1976.

3) Barnes, Broda Otto, and Charlotte W. Barnes. Heart Attack Rareness in thyroid-treated patients. Charles C Thomas Pub Ltd, 1972.

4) Barnes, Broda Otto, and Lawrence Galton. Hypothyroidism: The unsuspected illness. New York: Harper & Row, 1976.

5) Razvi, Salman, et al. "Levothyroxine treatment of subclinical hypothyroidism, fatal and nonfatal cardiovascular events, and mortality." Archives of internal medicine 172.10 (2012): 811–817.

6) Lev-Ran, Arye. "Thyroid hormones and prevention of atherosclerotic heart disease: an old-new hypothesis." Perspectives in biology and medicine 37.4 (1994): 486–494.

7) Jabbar, Avais, et al. "Thyroid hormones and cardiovascular disease." Nature Reviews Cardiology 14.1 (2017): 39.

8) Wren, James C. "Thyroid function and coronary atherosclerosis." Journal of the American Geriatrics Society 16.6 (1968): 696–704.

9) Wren, James C. "Symptomatic atherosclerosis: prevention or modification by treatment with desiccated thyroid." Journal of the American Geriatrics Society 19.1 (1971): 7–22.

10) Starr, Paul. "Atherosclerosis, hypothyroidism, and thyroid hormone therapy." Advances in lipid research. Vol. 16. Elsevier, 1978. 345–371.

11) Perrotta, Cristiana, et al. "The thyroid hormone triiodothyronine controls macrophage maturation and functions: protective role during inflammation." The American journal of pathology 184.1 (2014): 230–247.

12) De Vito, Paolo, et al. "Thyroid hormones as modulators of immune activities at the cellular level." Thyroid 21.8 (2011): 879–890.

13) Alamino, V. A., et al. "The thyroid hormone triiodothyronine reinvigorates dendritic cells and potentiates anti-tumor immunity." OncoImmunology 5.1 (2016): e1064579.

14) Schoenfeld, Philip S., et al. "Suppression of cell-mediated immunity in hypothyroidism." Southern medical journal 88.3 (1995): 347–349.

15) Pajkrt D, Doran JE, Koster F, et al. Antiinflammatory effects of reconstituted high-density lipoprotein during human endotoxemia. J Exp Med. 1996;184(5):1601–8.

16) Vreugdenhil AC, Rousseau CH, Hartung T, et al. Lipopolysaccharide (LPS)-binding protein mediates LPS detoxification by chylomicrons. J Immunol. 2003;170(3):1399–405.

17) Sandek A., Utchill S, Rauchhaus M. The endotoxin-lipoprotein hypothesis-an update. Arch Med Sci. 2007;3(4A):S81.

18) Chien JY, Jerng JS, Yu CJ, Yang PC. Low serum level of high-density lipoprotein cholesterol is a poor prognostic factor for severe sepsis. Crit Care Med. 2005;33(8):1688–93.

19) Åsvold, Bjørn O., et al. "Thyrotropin levels and risk of fatal coronary heart disease: the HUNT study." Archives of internal medicine 168.8 (2008): 855–860.

20) Åsvold, Bjørn O., et al. "The association between TSH within the reference range and serum lipid concentrations in a population-based study. The HUNT Study." European journal of endocrinology 156.2 (2007): 181–186.

21) Suh, Sunghwan, and Duk Kyu Kim. "Subclinical Hypothyroidism and Cardiovascular Disease." Endocrinology and Metabolism 30.3 (2015): 246.

22) Kvetny, J., et al. "Subclinical hypothyroidism is associated with a low-grade inflammation, increased triglyceride levels and predicts cardiovascular disease in males below 50 years." Clinical endocrinology 61.2 (2004): 232.

23) Hak, A. Elisabeth, et al. "Subclinical Hypothyroidism Is an Independent Risk Factor for Atherosclerosis and Myocardial Infarction in Elderly Women: The Rotterdam Study." Ann Intern Med 132 (2000): 270–278.

24) Imaizumi, Misa, et al. "Risk for ischemic heart disease and all-cause mortality in subclinical hypothyroidism." The Journal of Clinical Endocrinology & Metabolism 89.7 (2004): 3365–3370.

25) Rajagopalan, Viswanathan, et al. "Safe oral triiodo-l-thyronine therapy protects from post-infarct cardiac dysfunction and arrhythmias without cardiovascular adverse effects." PloS one 11.3 (2016): e0151413.

26) Tseng, Fen-Yu, et al. "Subclinical hypothyroidism is associated with increased risk for all-cause and cardiovascular mortality in adults." Journal of the American College of Cardiology 60.8 (2012): 730–737. Subclinical Hypothyroidism Associated With Increased Risk Cardiovascular Mortality Tseng FenYu J Amer Coll Cardiology 2012

27) Rhee, Connie M., et al. "Hypothyroidism and mortality among dialysis patients." Clinical Journal of the American Society of Nephrology (2012): CJN-06920712.

28) Razvi, Salman, et al. "The Incidence of Ischemic Heart Disease and Mortality in People with Subclinical Hypothyroidism: Reanalysis of the Whickham Survey Cohort." The Journal of clinical endocrinology and metabolism 95.4 (2010): 1734–1740.

29) Rodondi, Nicolas, et al. "Subclinical Hypothyroidism and the Risk of Coronary Heart Disease and Mortality." JAMA: the journal of the American Medical Association 304.12 (2010): 1365.

CHAPTER

21

Low Testosterone Could Be Killing You

IF YOU ARE A MALE, you might be interested to know that low testosterone is associated with increased mortality in observational studies. (1–3) In the first study from 2006, by Dr. Molly Shores, low testosterone was found to be associated with increased mortality among veterans. Eight hundred fifty-eight men were followed for 8 years. (1) A low testosterone level was defined as less than 250 ng/dL, and normal was defined as above 452 ng/dl. The low testosterone group had 35% mortality over 8 years compared to only 20% mortality for the normal testosterone group (hazard ratio, 1.88). (1)

The second study, published by Dr. Gail Laughlin in 2008, tracked nearly 800 men, 50 to 91 years old, living in California. Their testosterone level was measured at the beginning of the study, and their health was then tracked over the next 20 years. Low-testosterone symptoms reported by these men included decreased libido, erectile dysfunction, fatigue, loss of strength, decrease in bone density and decreased muscle mass. Also, these men tended to be overweight or obese, and at higher risk for cardiovascular disease and diabetes. Men with the lowest testosterone, below 241 total serum level, were 40% more likely to die. (2)

A third study, published by Dr. Chris Malkin in 2010 in *Heart,* showed that men with known coronary artery disease commonly had low testoster-one levels, which was associated with double the mortality rate of men with normal levels. (3) Nine hundred thirty males with coronary disease were followed for 7 years. Those with low testosterone had almost double the mortality Dr. Malkin says:

Excess mortality was noted in the androgen-deficient group compared with normal (21%) vs (12%). (3)

Postmenopausal Diabetic Women

A study published in 2011 *Diabetes Care* by Elisabeth Wehr from Graz, Austria, looked at testosterone levels in 875 postmenopausal women referred for coronary angiography who were followed for 7 years. The diabetic women with the highest quartile testosterone levels had a 60% reduction in all-cause and cardiovascular mortality compared to the lowest quartile. (5)

A similar study in older men referred for coronary angiography published by Dr. Elisabeth Lerchblaumin in 2012 in *Clinical Endocrinology* found that a combination of low free testosterone and low vitamin D predicts increased cardiovascular mortality. (6)

♦ ♦ ♦ ♦ ♦

♦ References for Chapter 21

1) Low Serum Testosterone and Mortality in Male Veterans Arch Intern Med. 2006;166:1660–1665 Molly M. Shores, MD; Alvin M. Matsumoto, MD; Kevin L. Sloan, MD; Daniel R. Kivlahan, PhD

2) Laughlin, Gail A., Elizabeth Barrett-Connor, and Jaclyn Bergstrom. "Low serum testosterone and mortality in older men." The Journal of Clinical Endocrinology & Metabolism 93.1 (2008): 68–75.

3) Malkin, Chris J., et al. "Low serum testosterone and increased mortality in men with coronary heart disease." Heart 96.22 (2010): 1821–1825.

4) deleted

5) Wehr, Elisabeth, et al. "Low free testosterone levels are associated with all-cause and cardiovascular mortality in postmenopausal diabetic women." Diabetes Care 34.8 (2011): 1771–1777.

6) Lerchbaum, Elisabeth, et al. "Combination of low free testosterone and low vitamin D predicts mortality in older men referred for coronary angiography." Clinical endocrinology 77.3 (2012): 475–483.

Testosterone Replacement Reduces Mortality

IF OBSERVATIONAL STUDIES SHOW LOW testosterone to be associated with increased mortality in males, the next question is: *What if these low-testosterone males are given testosterone replacement? Does this improve their survival and decrease the mortality rates?* The answer is YES in a number of studies.

Fifty-Percent Reduction in Mortality with Testosterone

A 2012 study by Dr. Molly Shores showed a 50% reduction in mortality in testosterone-treated males. Her study, published in the *Journal of Clinical Endocrinology & Metabolism*, followed 1,031 male veterans over the age of 40 for 4 years. All had low testosterone below 250, and a subgroup of 398 men were treated with testosterone replacement. At the end of 4 years, the testosterone-treated men had 10.3% mortality compared to 20.7% for the untreated men. (1) Testosterone supplementation reduced mortality by more than 50 per cent, a rather impressive result.

Larger Observational Study by Dr. Sharma

A retrospective observational study by Dr. Rishi Sharma in 83,000 male veterans with documented low testosterone levels over 6 years was published in 2015 in the *European Heart Journal*. (2) The mean age was 66 years. All-cause mortality for the testosterone-treated group was reduced by 56 per cent. Risk of heart attack was reduced 24%, and risk of stroke was reduced 36%.

(2) These results are impressive and in agreement with Dr. Molly Shore's 2012 study. Unfortunately, no calcium score data was reported. I would expect lower calcium scores in the testosterone-treated group.

Testosterone for Diabetic Males Reduces Mortality 50%

Dr. Vakkat Muraleedharan's 2013 study published in *European Journal of Endocrinology* showed a 50% reduction in mortality for testosterone-treated diabetic males. (10) The authors reported a mortality of 8.4% in diabetic men receiving testosterone over 6 years compared with 19.2% in untreated men. (9–11) This mortality reduction with testosterone far exceeds any other known drug treatment and is far superior to results of lipid-lowering drug trials. (15–17) What were the calcium scores in this study? We don't know, because they weren't done. Perhaps future studies will include calcium-score data, and if so, I would predict the testosterone group would show lower calcium scores.

Endocrine Society Recommends
Testosterone for Diabetic Males

About a quarter of diabetic men will have subnormal testosterone levels and inappropriately low LH and FSH, putting them at 200 to 300 per cent increased risk of cardiovascular mortality. (12) The Endocrine Society now recommends that diabetic men be tested for testosterone level and given testosterone replacement when found low. (14) (19) Testosterone replacement has found its place in mainstream medicine and is no longer controversial for diabetic males. (18–19)

♦ ♦ ♦ ♦ ♦

♦ References for Chapter 22

1) Shores, Molly M., et al. "Testosterone treatment and mortality in men with low testosterone levels." The Journal of Clinical Endocrinology & Metabolism 97.6 (2012): 2050–2058.

2) Sharma, Rishi, et al. "Normalization of testosterone level is associated with reduced incidence of myocardial infarction and mortality in men." European Heart Journal (2015): ehv346.

3) deleted

4) Dandona, Paresh, and Sandeep Dhindsa. "Update: hypogonadotropic hypogonadism in type 2 diabetes and obesity." The Journal of Clinical Endocrinology & Metabolism 96.9 (2011): 2643–2651.

5) Guidelines on Male Hypogonadism Dohle 2015 European Association of Urology.

6) Friedrich, Nele, et al. "Improved prediction of all-cause mortality by a combination of serum total testosterone and insulin-like growth factor I in adult men." Steroids 77.1 (2012): 52–58.

7) Cunningham, Glenn R., and Shivani M. Toma. "Why is androgen replacement in males controversial?." The Journal of Clinical Endocrinology & Metabolism 96.1 (2011): 38–52.

8) Swerdloff, Ronald, and Christina Wang. "Testosterone treatment of older men—why are controversies created?." (2011): 62–65.

9) Muraleedharan, Vakkat, Hazel Marsh, and Hugh Jones. "Low testosterone predicts increased mortality and testosterone replacement therapy improves survival in men with type 2 diabetes." (2011).

10) Muraleedharan, Vakkat, et al. "Testosterone deficiency is associated with increased risk of mortality and testosterone replacement improves survival in men with type 2 diabetes." European Journal of Endocrinology 169.6 (2013): 725–733.

11) Muraleedharan, Vakkat, and T. Hugh Jones. "Testosterone and the metabolic syndrome." Therapeutic advances in endocrinology and metabolism 1.5 (2010): 207–223.

12) Dandona, Paresh, and Sandeep Dhindsa. "Update: hypogonadotropic hypogonadism in type 2 diabetes and obesity." The Journal of Clinical Endocrinology & Metabolism 96.9 (2011): 2643–2651.

13) Kapoor, Dheeraj, and T. Hugh Jones. "Androgen deficiency as a predictor of metabolic syndrome in aging men." Drugs & aging 25.5 (2008): 357–369.

14) Society for Endocrinology Media Release Wednesday 13 April 2011.

15) Kjekshus, John, Terje R. Pedersen, and Scandinavian Simvastatin Survival Study Group. "Reducing the risk of coronary events: evidence from the Scandinavian Simvastatin Survival Study (4S)." The American journal of cardiology 76.9 (1995): 64C-68C.

16) Pedersen, Terje R., et al. "Lipoprotein changes and reduction in the incidence of major coronary heart disease events in the Scandinavian Simvastatin Survival Study (4S)." Circulation 97.15 (1998): 1453–1460.

17) Marschner, I. C. "Long-term intervention with pravastatin in ischemic disease (LIPID) study: Long-term risk stratification for survivors of acute coronary syndromes: Results from the long-term intervention with pravastatin in ischemic disease (LIPID) study. LIPID Study Investigators." J Am Coll Cardiol 38 (2001): 56–63.

18) Jones, T. Hugh, R. Quinton, and A. Ullah. "Every obese male with type 2 diabetes should be screened for hypogonadism." Practical Diabetes 28.1 (2011): 14.

19) Bhasin, Shalender, et al. "Testosterone therapy in men with androgen deficiency syndromes: an Endocrine Society clinical practice guideline." The Journal of Clinical Endocrinology & Metabolism 95.6 (2010): 2536–2559.

20) Anderson, Jeffrey L., et al. "Impact of testosterone replacement therapy on myocardial infarction, stroke, and death in men with low testosterone concentrations in an integrated health care system." The American journal of cardiology 117.5 (2016): 794–799.

21) Saad, Farid, et al. "Testosterone deficiency and testosterone treatment in older men." Gerontology 63.2 (2017): 144–156.

22) Morgentaler, Abraham, et al. "Testosterone therapy and cardiovascular risk: advances and controversies." Mayo Clinic Proceedings. Vol. 90. No. 2. Elsevier, 2015.

Testosterone Therapy, Coronary Plaque, and Calcium Score

JIM IS A RETIRED 72-YEAR-OLD who had a stent placed a few years ago for coronary artery disease. Jim had low testosterone on his initial lab panel and has been using topical testosterone for a few years now. Last week, his primary care doctors told him that he should not be taking testosterone, as a new study shows testosterone increases atherosclerotic plaque formation. This was the *JAMA* 2017 study by Dr. Budoff, which reported the testosterone group has increased non-calcified plaque compared to the placebo group. (1) Paradoxically, the testosterone group did better, with less progression of coronary calcium score compared to the placebo group. There were no adverse cardiac events in either group over the one year of observation.

Alarm Bells Go Off

Medical writer Eric Barnes declares, *"Testosterone treatment raises levels of heart plaque."* (21) Marlene Buskos declares *"Atherosclerosis Speeds Up in Older Men on Testosterone"* (24) Can this be true? Are these statements correct or are they wrong? Below, we will take a critical look at the 2017 *JAMA* Budoff study.

A Critical Look at the Budoff Testosterone Study

Study details: About 140 males in their early 70s with known coronary artery disease and calcium score above 300 were randomized to receive testosterone or placebo. They were then followed for 12 months. Many of the men had obesity, hypertension, hyperlipidemia, and diabetes. The men were studied with baseline and annual CAT scan with calcium score and coronary artery imaging with IV contrast.

The calcium score results showed the testosterone group had a mean increase of 53 units, compared to 118 for the placebo-treated group. However, the authors reported no significant difference in calcium score for testosterone vs placebo.

Problems with the study: Number one, if this had been a truly randomized study, the starting calcium scores for the treatment and placebo groups should have been similar. They were quite different (255 vs. 454), suggesting some problem with randomization.

Second Problem: It is well known that heavily calcified arteries with high calcium score, as in the placebo group (454), cause streak artifact and technical difficulties obtaining accurate readings for noncalcified plaque. The calcification is extremely dense on the CAT scan, making exact quantification of soft plaque prone to technical error.

Here is a quote from Dr. Z. Sun in 2016 in "Coronary CT angiography in coronary artery disease" in the Australasian Medical Journal (2):

> *"Extensive coronary artery calcification (coronary calcium score >400) still limits the diagnostic accuracy of CCTA in CAD, in particular, reducing the sensitivity to some extent due to high rate of false positive results. ". . . . clinical value of CCTA is controversial." (2) (Note CCTA = Coronary CT Angiography, CAD= Coronary Artery Disease)*

Third problem: The clinical relevance of the coronary artery calcium score is well established and in routine use. The clinical relevance of noncalcified plaque is controversial and not in routine clinical use.

Testosterone and Calcium Score Studies

We have good calcium score data from a 2015 study by Dr. Shehzad Basaria published in *JAMA* in 2015. The annual rate of change of coronary calcium was significantly lower in the testosterone group non-statin users.

(22) Dr. Basaria says the annual rate of change was significantly lower in the testosterone-treated group (non-statin users).

However, in a post hoc exploratory analysis of observed data restricted to statin non-users, the annual rate of change in coronary artery calcium was significantly lower in the testosterone group than in the placebo group (mean difference, −30.1)." (22)

This 2015 Basaria Calcium Score Data is hard to find and was presented in Supplementary Figure 6 Calcium score statin non-users. Dr. Basaria speculated that perhaps statin drug use masks the benefits of testosterone for reducing calcium score progression. This is possible, since statin drugs actually stimulate arterial calcification by inhibiting Vitamin K (see chapter 4), as discussed by Dr. Haruumi Okuyama in his 2015 paper in Expert Review of Clinical Pharmacology. (7) As discussed in chapter 4, Dr. Edward A. Gill reported statin drugs performed no better than placebo for calcium score, a disappointment for mainstream cardiology.

Calcium Score Inverse with Testosterone Level

Dr. Park found an inverse relationship between serum testosterone and calcium score. (11) Drs. Lai and Khazai independently confirmed Dr. Park's findings of an inverse relationship between testosterone and coronary artery calcium score. (35,36) They both found that low testosterone is associated with higher calcium scores.

The Robust Predictive Ability of Coronary Calcium Score

The coronary calcium score as discussed in previous chapters is a very useful clinical tool currently in wide use to predict coronary risk. On the other hand, CAT-scan detection of non-calcified plaque as done in the 2017 Matt Budoff study has not been clinically useful and is not a good method for predicting coronary risk. The most likely reason for this is the increased arterial calcification in patients with advanced disease masking the soft plaque, creating technical artifacts. Here is a quote from Dr. Stephan Achenbach in 2010 from "Imaging of Coronary Atherosclerosis by Computed Tomography":

So far, the available clinical data are not sufficient to draw specific conclusions as to the risk–benefit ratio of contrast-enhanced coronary CTA (computed tomography angiography) for risk prediction, especially for asymptomatic individuals. Hence, CTA is currently not recommended for risk stratification purposes. (4)

Rather than used as a standalone tool, CAT scan coronary angiography for detection of non-calcified plaque is useful as an add-on to the calcium score test to improve discriminatory value. (3) If the calcium score is low (or zero), presence of complete obstruction or high-grade stenosis on the CAT angiogram adds significant information which changes the prognosis. However, CAT-scan coronary calcium score is the best predictor of non-calcified plaque in patients with low calcium score. (28)

Another red warning flag: Dr. Matt Budoff's 2017 study concludes that testosterone increases plaque formation in men with coronary artery disease. However, Dr. Budoff reports in his study, over 12 months of testosterone use, there were no cardiovascular events. If testosterone was as bad as he says, where are the worsening ischemic events, myocardial infarctions, and increased mortality in the testosterone-treated group? There were none.

The conclusions of the 2017 JAMA study by Dr. Budoff contradict 40 years of previous medical studies on the effects of testosterone on the cardiovascular system. According to Dr. A. Traish in 2016 (5)

There is no credible evidence to indicate that Testosterone therapy increases the risk of CVD (cardiovascular disease). On the contrary, Testosterone therapy may be protective. . . . Testosterone therapy has been used as early as 1940s with no reported adverse effects on the CV (cardiovascular) system. (5) . . . Recent observational, registry studies, clinical trials, and meta-analyses, all revealed no increase in CV (cardiovascular) risks in men receiving Testosterone therapy. (6)

Dr. Budoff's 2017 *JAMA* study suggests that testosterone worsens coronary artery disease in males by causing more plaque formation, more myocardial ischemia, more arterial occlusion, more myocardial infarction, and increased mortality from heart disease. As we can see clearly from a real-life experience at two urology clinics over 8 years treating 77 males with known coronary artery disease, none of this actually happens as reported by Dr. Haider in 2016. (8) No cardiovascular events were reported in the testosterone-treated group over 8 years, and various cardiovascular risk parameters were improved. Here is a quote from Dr. Haider in 2016 describing the effect of 8 years of follow-up in 77 testosterone-treated males with underlying heart disease:

> *Over 8 years, the men experienced weight loss (from 114 kg to 91 kg), decreased waist circumference (112 cm to 99 cm), decreased BMI from 37 to 29. Cardio-metabolic parameters such as lipid profile, glycemic control, blood pressure, heart rate, and pulse pressure all improved significantly and sustainably. No patient suffered a major adverse cardiovascular event during the full observation time. Testosterone therapy. . . . may be effective as an add-on treatment for secondary prevention of cardiovascular events in testosterone-deficient men with a history of cardiovascular disease. (8)*

What were the calcium scores on these men in the Haider study? We don't know, because they were not obtained. I would expect the calcium score data would have shown slower progression in the testosterone group. Perhaps future studies will answer this question.

Younger Men Without Heart Disease

If testosterone increases plaque formation in a clinically significant way, as Dr. Budoff is suggesting, then this should result in increased myocardial ischemic events, myocardial infarction, and death in healthy males of any age who receive testosterone treatment. In reviewing registries for 20,000 males receiving testosterone therapy, with an average age of 46, Dr. Robert Tan had this to say:

> *There was no evidence of worsening preexisting MI or stroke in patients treated with testosterone. (9)*

Dr. Yeap found that LOW testosterone levels in older men were predictive of increased stroke and Transient Ischemic Attacks (TIAs) (37) If testosterone is an evil hormone that makes men die of coronary artery disease, then surely men with low testosterone should be protected from this evil drug, and men with high testosterone should succumb to its adverse effects. Studies show that just the opposite is true. (11–13)(38) In Dr. Haider's 2016 review of the available medical literature, we find:

> *Mortality in men with Testosterone Deficiency was reduced subsequent to Testosterone Therapy. Molly Shores et al. demonstrated that mortality in Testosterone-treated men was 10.3% compared with 20.7% in untreated hypogonadal men. Muraleedharan demonstrated, in hypogonadal men with type 2 diabetes mellitus, reduced mortality of 8.4% in men receiving Testosterone Therapy compared with 19.2% in untreated men. These findings are consistent with several studies summarized by Morgentaler. Cardiovascular benefits of Testosterone Therapy have been shown in interventional studies, including benefits in men with congestive heart failure, cardiac ischemia/angina, including a reduction in carotid intima–media thickness. Most studies identified an inverse association between serum Testosterone concentration and all-cause or CV mortality. (8)*

If testosterone is the evil drug that worsens plaque formation in men with coronary artery disease, then one would expect men with angina would be made worse by testosterone. The opposite is true. Numerous studies show testosterone improves ischemic threshold in men with angina and improves quality of life (14–15)

Dr. Andrew Elagizi published his review of the medical literature in the 2018 *Mayo Clinic Proceedings*. Dr. Elagizi says the medical literature is contradictory on testosterone use in cardiovascular disease.

> *Testosterone levels may directly cause (or prevent) Coronary artery disease and Cardiovascular events, or testosterone levels may simply be a marker of overall quality of health and have no direct effect on Coronary artery disease and Cardiovascular events at all. (39)*

Dr. Elagizi's comments may be on the mark. Perhaps the "quality of health" is one of numerous conditions causing HPA dysfunction. Obesity, metabolic syndrome, and diabetes are all associated with leaky gut and low-level endotoxemia, HPA dysfunction, and low testosterone. (42) Perhaps this is the "marker of quality of health" Dr. Elagizi is referring to.(Note: HPA Dysfunction = Hypothalamic Pituitary Dysfunction)

Hypothalamic Dysfunction in Low Testosterone Males Is Common

In post-menopausal females, laboratory studies invariably demonstrate high LH and FSH (LH=leutinizing hormone, FSH = follicle stimulating hormone) These are hallmarks of ovarian failure and definite evidence the female patient is post-menopausal. In males, a similar elevation in LH and FSH is reported for aging males with an inflection point on the charts around age 70, after which a steeper increase in LH is observed. However quite surprisingly, many symptomatic males in the 40–70 age group presenting for testosterone treatment have LH and FSH values lower than expected, suggesting HPA dysfunction from underlying health problems, as Dr. Andrew Elagizi has so astutely mentioned. (43–47) One of these underlying health problems is obesity, a main feature of metabolic syndrome, known to cause HPA dysfunction and low testosterone. (47)

Leaky Gut, Hypothalamic Dysfunction, High Calcium Score

Disruption of the gut barrier with increased permeability, also, as we have seen, called leaky gut, has been implicated in diabetes, metabolic syndrome, obesity, atherosclerosis, and neurodegenerative disorders. Leaky gut causes low-level endotoxemia and atherosclerosis, as discussed in chapter 12 on atherosclerotic plaque as infected biofilm. If low-level endotoxemia from leaky gut is causing HPA dysfunction and low testosterone, then the correct treatment is to address leaky gut, not testosterone replacement. For this reason, in younger males with HPA dysfunction from leaky gut, we avoid using testosterone and instead may use other agents which stimulate endogenous testosterone production such as clomiphene, originally FDA approved as a fertility drug for women. Clomiphene is commonly used off-label in males to stimulate testosterone production. Because of possible visual adverse side effects, clomiphene is usually used short term or on a schedule with off-days included. Alternatively, HCG (human chorionic gonadotropin, an LH analog) may be used to stimulate endogenous testosterone production, while addressing the leaky gut issues.

Conclusion

The 2017 *JAMA* Budoff study contradicts 40 years of published data on testosterone and cardiovascular disease. Real world data from two Urology Clinics treating males with cardiovascular disease with testosterone for 8 years shows the striking benefit of testosterone treatment for males with known cardiovascular disease.

♦　♦　♦　♦　♦

◆ References for Chapter 23

1) Budoff, Matthew J., et al. "Testosterone treatment and coronary artery plaque volume in older men with low testosterone." Jama 317.7 (2017): 708–716.

2) Sun, Zhonghua. "Coronary CT angiography in coronary artery disease: Opportunities and challenges." Australasian Medical Journal 9.5 (2016). Coronary CT angiography in coronary artery disease Sun Zhonghua Australasian Medical Journal 2016

3) Al-Mallah, Mouaz H., et al. "Does coronary CT angiography improve risk stratification over coronary calcium scoring in symptomatic patients with suspected coronary artery disease? Results from the prospective multicenter international CONFIRM registry." European Heart Journal–Cardiovascular Imaging 15.3 (2013): 267–274.

4) Achenbach, Stephan, and Paolo Raggi. "Imaging of coronary atherosclerosis by computed tomography." European heart journal (2010): ehq150.

5) Traish, Abdulmaged. "Testosterone therapy men testosterone deficiency : Are we beyond the point of no return?." Investigative and Clinical Urology 57.6 (2016): 384–400.

6) Traish, Abdulmaged M. "Testosterone therapy in men with testosterone deficiency: are the benefits and cardiovascular risks real or imagined?" American Journal of Physiology-Regulatory, Integrative and Comparative Physiology. Vol. 311. No. 3. American Physiological Society, 2016.

7) Okuyama, Harumi, et al. "Statins stimulate atherosclerosis and heart failure: pharmacological mechanisms." Expert review of clinical pharmacology 8.2 (2015): 189–199.

8) Haider, Ahmad, et al. "Men with testosterone deficiency and a history of cardiovascular diseases benefit from long-term testosterone therapy: observational, real-life data from a registry study." Vascular health and risk management 12 (2016): 251.

9) Tan, Robert S., Kelly R. Cook, and William G. Reilly. "Myocardial Infarction and Stroke Risk in Young Healthy Men Treated with Injectable Testosterone." (2015). Myocardial Infarction and Stroke Risk in Young Healthy Men Treated with Injectable Testosterone Tan Robert Kelly Cook 2015

10) Kelly, Daniel M., and T. Hugh Jones. "Testosterone and cardiovascular risk in men." Cardiovascular Issues in Endocrinology. Vol. 43. Karger Publishers, 2014. 1–20.

11) Park, Byoung-Jin, et al. "Inverse relationship between bioavailable testosterone and subclinical coronary artery calcification in non-obese Korean men." Asian journal of andrology 14.4 (2012): 612–615.

12) Morgentaler, Abraham, Allison Feibus, and Neil Baum. "Testosterone and cardiovascular disease–the controversy and the facts." Postgraduate medicine 127.2 (2015): 159–165

13) Morgentaler, Abraham. "Testosterone deficiency and cardiovascular mortality." Asian journal of andrology 17.1 (2015): 26.

14) English, Katherine M., et al. "Low-dose transdermal testosterone therapy improves angina threshold in men with chronic stable angina." Circulation 102.16 (2000): 1906–1911.

15) Malkin, C. J., et al. "Testosterone replacement in hypogonadal men with angina improves ischaemic threshold and quality of life." Heart 90.8 (2004): 871–876.

16) Khaw, Kay-Tee, et al. "Endogenous testosterone and mortality due to all causes, cardiovascular disease, and cancer in men." Circulation 116.23 (2007): 2694–2701.

17) Gururani, Kunal, John Jose, and Paul V. George. "Testosterone as a marker of coronary artery disease severity in middle-aged males." Indian Heart Journal 68 (2016): S16-S20.

18) Li, Z. B., et al. "Testosterone therapy improves cardiac function of male rats with right heart failure." Zhonghua nan ke xue= National journal of andrology 15.11 (2009): 994–1000.

19) Malkin, C. J., et al. "Testosterone therapy in men with moderate severity heart failure: a double-blind randomized placebo controlled trial." European heart journal 27.1 (2006): 57. Testosterone therapy men moderate heart failure randomized trial Malkin C J European heart journal 2006

20) Pugh, P. J., et al. "Testosterone treatment for men with chronic heart failure." Heart 90.4 (2004): 446–447. Testosterone treatment for men with chronic heart failure Pugh PJ Heart 2004

21) Testosterone treatment raises levels of heart plaque By Eric Barnes, AuntMinnie.com staff writer

22) Basaria, Shehzad, et al. "Effects of testosterone administration for 3 years on subclinical atherosclerosis progression in older men with low or low-normal testosterone levels: a randomized clinical trial." Jama 314.6 (2015): 570–581.

23) Coronary Artery Calcium Scoring Can Help Guide Statin Therapy Matthew J. Budoff, MD January 14, 2016

24) Atherosclerosis Speeds Up in Older Men on Testosterone: T Trial by Marlene Busko February 24, 2017

25) Snyder, Peter J., et al. "The Testosterone Trials: The Design of Seven Coordinated Trials to Determine if Testosterone Treatment Benefits Elderly Men." Clinical trials (London, England) 11.3: 362.

26) Handelsman, David J. "Testosterone and male aging: faltering hope for rejuvenation." Jama 317.7 (2017): 699–701.

27) deleted

28) Tam, Lori M., et al. "Absolute coronary artery calcium score is the best predictor of non-calcified plaque involvement in patients with low calcium scores (1e100)." Atherosclerosis 230.7 (2013): 6e79.

29) Yoo, Dong Hyun, et al. "Significance of noncalcified coronary plaque in asymptomatic subjects with low coronary artery calcium score: assessment with coronary computed tomography angiography." The international journal of cardiovascular imaging 27.1 (2011): 27–35.

30) Naya, Masanao, et al. "Quantitative relationship between the extent and morphology of coronary atherosclerotic plaque and downstream myocardial perfusion." Journal of the American College of Cardiology 58.17 (2011): 1807–1816.

31) Gaur, Sara, et al. "Coronary plaque quantification and fractional flow reserve by coronary computed tomography angiography identify ischaemia-causing lesions." European heart journal 37.15 (2016): 1220–1227.

32) Bauer, Ralf W., et al. "Noncalcified atherosclerotic plaque burden at coronary CT angiography: a better predictor of ischemia at stress myocardial perfusion imaging than calcium score and stenosis severity." American Journal of Roentgenology 193.2 (2009): 410–418.

33) Mathur, Atish, et al. "Long-term benefits of testosterone replacement therapy on angina threshold and atheroma in men." European Journal of Endocrinology 161.3 (2009): 443–449.

34) Toma, Mustafa, et al. "Testosterone Supplementation in Heart Failure Clinical Perspective." Circulation: Heart Failure 5.3 (2012): 315–321.

35) Lai, Jiangtao, et al. "Low serum testosterone level was associated with extensive coronary artery calcification in elderly male patients with stable coronary artery disease." Coronary artery disease 26.5 (2015): 437–441.

36) Khazai, Bahram, et al. "Association of endogenous testosterone with subclinical atherosclerosis in men: the mult-ethnic study of atherosclerosis." Clinical endocrinology (2016).

37) Yeap, Bu B., et al. "Lower testosterone levels predict incident stroke and transient ischemic attack in older men." The Journal of Clinical Endocrinology & Metabolism 94.7 (2009): 2353–2359.

38) Cheetham, T. Craig, et al. "Association of testosterone replacement with cardiovascular outcomes among men with androgen deficiency." JAMA internal medicine 177.4 (2017): 491–499.

39) Elagizi, Andrew, Tobias S. Köhler, and Carl J. Lavie. "testosterone and Cardiovascular Health." Mayo Clinic Proceedings. Vol. 93. No. 1. Elsevier, 2018.

40) Webb, Carolyn M., Collins, Peter, 'Role of Testosterone in the Treatment of Cardiovascular Disease," European Cardiology Review 2017;12(2):83–7..

41) Glueck, Charles J., et al. "Thrombophilia in 67 patients with thrombotic events after starting testosterone therapy." Clinical and Applied Thrombosis/Hemostasis 22.6 (2016): 548–553.

42) Dach, Jeffrey. "Gut-Brain: Major Depressive Disorder, Hypothalamic Dysfunction, and High Calcium Score Associated With Leaky Gut." Alternative therapies in health and medicine 21 (2015): 10.

43) Kaufman, Jean M., and Alex Vermeulen. "The Decline of Androgen Levels in Elderly Men and Its Clinical and Therapeutic Implications." Endocrine Reviews 26.6: 833–876.

44) Wu, Frederick CW, et al. "Hypothalamic-pituitary-testicular axis disruptions in older men are differentially linked to age and modifiable risk factors: the European Male Aging Study." The Journal of Clinical Endocrinology & Metabolism 93.7 (2008): 2737–2745.

45) Morley, John E., et al. "Longitudinal changes in testosterone, luteinizing hormone, and follicle-stimulating hormone in healthy older men." Metabolism-Clinical and Experimental 46.4 (1997): 410–413.

46) KORENMAN, STANLEY G., et al. "Secondary hypogonadism in older men: its relation to impotence." The Journal of Clinical Endocrinology & Metabolism 71.4 (1990): 963–969.

47) Camacho, EM1, et al. "Age-associated changes in hypothalamic-pituitary-testicular function in middle-aged and older men are modified by weight change and lifestyle factors: longitudinal results from the European Male Ageing Study." European Journal of Endocrinology 168.3 (2013): 445–455.

A Man with Progressive Coronary Artery Disease Unresponsive to Statins

SIXTY-TWO-YEAR-OLD JIM JUST HAD HIS third cardiac stent. A year ago, he noticed a "tight feeling" in his chest radiating to his throat and was rushed to the ER, where doctors found he was having a heart attack. A coronary angiogram showed extensive coronary artery disease with irregular plaque formation.

Progressive Coronary Artery Plaque in Spite of Low Cholesterol

Jim had been taking a statin drug for 12 years. His cholesterol level had been driven down to 140 by his "top cardiologist," who prescribed a hefty dose of a statin anti-cholesterol drug. In spite of the lowest cholesterol level on the planet, Jim's heart disease progressed relentlessly, with worsening calcium scores, worsening angiograms, and worsening symptoms of chest pain. His disease progression was obviously not caused by an elevated cholesterol level. For a discussion of how elevated cholesterol is NOT the Cause of Heart Disease, see chapter 25, on familial hypercholesterolemia. These are the elderly patients with extremely high cholesterol, yet no heart disease, disproving the cholesterol theory of heart disease. In this scenario, reducing cholesterol levels with drugs is ill-advised.

Doctors Advise Jim to Stop Testosterone

Jim had been taking topical testosterone for the past 5 years, but recently stopped it on the advice of his cardiologist, who pointed a finger and said, *"You should stop the testosterone. . . . The testosterone is bad for your heart and probably caused your heart attack. "Jim* came to see me for a second opinion.

Jim's Doctor Is Right About That

Jim's doctor is right in that a number of recent studies have shown a small increase in heart attack rate in men starting testosterone. This is caused by increased hematocrit (red blood cell count) and increased iron stores, which thicken the blood and make it more susceptible to blood clot formation—all risk factors for heart attack. The simple solution is to monitor blood count and iron levels and donate blood at the blood bank every 4 to 6 weeks to reduce iron and red cells.

Bio-identical Hormones for Prevention and Reversal of Heart Disease

In this article we will revisit the role of the testosterone and estradiol in the prevention and reversal of heart disease, looking at the latest research. First, let's try to answer the following question: *Is low testosterone a risk factor for heart disease, and is a normal testosterone level protective of heart disease?*

Here we assume red cell count and iron levels are kept under control with monthly trips to the blood bank, so there is no short-term increase in heart attack rate from hypercoagulability, as noted in a few recent studies of men started on testosterone.

Low Testosterone is Predictive for Increased Mortality from Heart Disease

If testosterone were causative of heart disease, one would expect men with high testosterone to have more heart disease and men with low testosterone to have less heart disease. This is exactly the opposite of four major studies showing that men with low testosterone have both increased all-cause mortality and increased heart disease mortality. (1–4)

Testosterone Levels in Men with Heart Disease

A recent study by Dr. Malkin looked at testosterone levels in men with known underlying heart disease. He showed that low testosterone is common in men with underlying heart disease and this is associated with almost double the mortality rate. (5) Again, these findings suggest that higher testosterone is protective and prevents progression of heart disease. The assumption that testosterone causes progression of atherosclerosis plaque has been shown to be false. (6)(8)

Animal Studies on Mechanism of Protection

A number of elegant animal studies have elucidated the mechanism by which testosterone is protective of heart disease. A 1999 study by Alex Andersen showed that testosterone reduced aortic atherosclerosis in rabbits. (10) Castrated rabbits had low testosterone levels and doubled the aortic atherosclerosis plaque formation, suggesting that testosterone has a strong preventive effect on male atherosclerosis. In the groups receiving testosterone or DHEA, they found marked inhibition of atherosclerosis compared with placebo. The mechanism was not clearly defined. They speculated on a non-lipid mediated mechanism, possibly related to aromatase conversion of testosterone to estrogen. (10)

Mouse Model: It's Really the Estrogen That's Protective

In a well-designed 2001 study published in *Proceedings of the National Academy of Sciences,* Nathan et al. used a mouse model of accelerated atherosclerosis to show that testosterone inhibits atherosclerosis through its conversion to estrogen by the aromatase enzyme. Similar protection from atherosclerosis was obtained by administering estradiol. In addition, blocking conversion of testosterone to estradiol with the aromatase inhibitor, anastrazole, eliminated the protective effect, and these animals had progressive atherosclerosis. (11) Dr. Nathan says:

> *Testosterone attenuates early atherogenesis most likely by being converted to estrogens by the enzyme aromatase expressed in the vessel wall. (11)*

The results of this study suggest that men with heart disease should not drive down estrogen levels with aromatase inhibitors.

Genetically Altered Mouse Model Provides Answers

These findings were confirmed by Joanne Nettleship in a 2007 study published in *Circulation* using the Tfm genetically modified mouse. This mouse is genetically altered to have a defective androgen receptor. In these mice, testosterone cannot work through its normal pathway, since there is no receptor. In spite of the lack of androgen receptor, Nettleship found that testosterone replacement in these mice attenuated atherosclerotic changes (fatty streak formation), suggesting the protective effect of testosterone was independent of the testosterone receptor. The authors concluded that the protective benefits of testosterone were through aromatase conversion to estradiol, and then via the estrogen receptor pathways. (12)

Dr. Nettleship's findings were confirmed by Burghardt in a Nov 2010 study published in Endocrinology that used' "ARKO" mice, genetically modified to "knock out" the androgen receptor, modified to be apoE-deficient, to accelerate atherosclerosis. The authors showed that testosterone therapy administered to the ARKO mice inhibited atherosclerosis. However, inhibition of atherosclerosis was more profound in the wild-type mice that still had intact androgen receptors. The authors concluded the mechanism of protection of testosterone was due to both mechanisms, through the androgen receptor as well as through aromatase conversion to estradiol. (13)

These genetically modified mouse studies suggest that testosterone's cardio-protective benefits are due to conversion to estrogen, and that estrogen is the cardio-protective agent. Both estrogen and testosterone are bio-identical hormones. Clearly, the message here is that testosterone replacement therapy should be an important part of any heart-disease prevention program in those patients who have low testosterone levels.

Defective Estrogen Receptor in Males with Coronary Artery Disease

In 1997, Dr. Sudhir reports a case of premature coronary artery disease associated with a mutation in the estrogen receptor gene in a thirty-one-year-old male. (32) This patient was insensitive to the effects of estrogen. The patient's lipid profile showed a very low total cholesterol of 130, yet his calcium score of 47 was very high for his age (95 percentile).

Why Do Men Have More Heart Disease Than Women?

Men and women are quite different when it comes to heart disease. Men have more than twice the risk of dying from coronary disease than women. (14) In women, coronary artery disease develops on average 10 years later than in men. (15) Could higher levels of estrogen (estradiol) in women explain the protection enjoyed by women?

Dr. Dongqi Xing from the University of Alabama would say, yes of course estrogen is protective. In a 2009 article, Dr. Xing names a number of mechanisms by which estradiol protects both men and women from heart disease. He says:

Estrogens have antiinflammatory and vasoprotective effects. Natural endogenous estrogen 17β-estradiol (bioidentical) has been shown to cause rapid endothelium-independent dilation of coronary arteries of men and women, to augment endothelium-dependent relaxation of

human coronary arteries, and improve endothelial function . . . Obser-
vational studies have shown substantial benefit (50% reduction in heart
disease) of hormone therapy in women who choose to use menopausal
hormones. (15)

Estrogen is Protective of Heart Disease

A 2010 study in *European Heart* by Kitamura et al. compared male to female heart attack rates. They found 61% fewer heart attacks in women of reproductive age with high estrogen levels compared to males of the same age. The authors conclude that estrogen confers cardio-protective benefits. (16)

A review of the "Nurse Health Study" published in the 2000 *Annals* showed a 40% reduction in heart disease in hormone replacement users and that *"postmenopausal hormone use decreases risk for major coronary events."* (17–18)

Mainstream Treatments for Coronary Artery Disease

There are three mainstream treatments for coronary artery disease:

1) Surgery with coronary artery bypass

2) Balloon angioplasty with stenting

3) Medical therapy with drugs such as calcium-channel blockers, nitro-glycerine vasodilators, ACE inhibitors, and beta blockers.

Which one of these treatment modalities confers the most benefit? The answer is: None of them.

Medical Management with Drugs Provides the Same Benefit as Cardiac Angioplasty, Stenting, or Bypass

Eleven randomized studies reviewed 3,000 patients with stable coronary artery disease. Treatment with angioplasty and stenting showed the same mortality rate and heart attack rate as drug treatment, also known as medical management. Both offer the same benefit. (19)(20)

The MASS II study published in 2007 in *Circulation* showed that medical management offered similar outcomes to stent or bypass. (21) A troubling fact remains that after all these studies have been completed, there is no conclusive evidence that a coronary artery bypass graft or coronary stent is superior to medical therapy with drugs for treating multivessel coronary artery disease with stable angina and preserved ventricular function. (21) Sorano attempts to sort out the fine points of selecting between treatment modalities in her 2009 report. (22)

How Can Drugs Provide the Same Outcome as Surgery or Stenting?

Now we have an important question to ask. *How is it possible that the humble country doctor with a few drugs can provide similar outcomes as the high and mighty cardiac surgeon and the interventional cardiologist? How can drug treatment do as well or better than the cardiac stent or surgical bypass procedure?*

I suggest the answer resides in the phenomenon known as "collateral vessel formation." The heart has the ability to grow new blood vessels that provide blood flow around the blocked artery. Medical treatment gives the heart time to grow new collateral vessels. The key to understanding this new vessel formation is the endothelial progenitor cell, also known as the EPC, a special type of stem cell found in the bone marrow that circulates to injured myocardium, where it promotes local angiogenesis, the making of new blood vessels. (23)

Turning on the Endothelial Progenitor Cell: How to Do It?

Telomers are small pieces of our DNA which control aging. As our telomeres shorten with each stage of cell replication, this determines how fast we age. Estrogen serves as an anti-aging therapy by preventing the telomeres from shortening. Recent research shows that estrogen activates the telomeres on endothelial progenitor cells (EPC) and improves the EPC functional capacity. (24) Another study showed reduced numbers of EPC cells in the peripheral blood of men with low testosterone levels. (25)

Estradiol Enhances Recovery After Myocardial Infarction: Collateral Vessels

An elegant study published by Isakura in 2006 *Circulation* used a mouse model in which myocardial infarction was induced by ligation of the left coronary artery. The estradiol-treated mice showed increased circulating EPCs and greater capillary density in the recovering myocardium. This indicates enhanced recovery in the estradiol-treated mice by regrowth of collateral vessels. (26–28) An Italian study by Chiara Bolego showed that the cardio-protective benefits of estrogen could be duplicated with an estrogen-receptor drug called PPT. They found that

> *myocardial ischemia-reperfusion injury was exacerbated by ovariectomy (which reduced estrogen levels). This injury returned to baseline following treatment with estrogen-like drug PPT. (29)*

The protective effects were linked to increased levels of EPCs. (29)

Recent research shows the cardio-protective benefits of the bio-identical hormones testosterone and estrogen. Testosterone benefit appears mediated by conversion to estradiol via the aromatase enzyme. Estradiol's benefits appear related to activation of endothelial progenitor cells, which invoke new collateral circulation in areas of injury.

EECP (Extra-Corporeal Counterpulsation)

Another treatment modality called EECP (Extra-Corporeal Counterpulsation) should be mentioned here. This also invokes new collateral vessels by activating EPCs—the stem cells—using counterpulsating blood pressure cuffs placed over the extremities. (33–36)

♦ ♦ ♦ ♦ ♦

♦ References for Chapter 24

1) Shores MM, Moceri VM, Gruenewald DA, et al. Low testosterone is associated with decreased function and increased mortality risk: a preliminary study of men in a geriatric rehabilitation unit. J Am Geriatr Soc 2004;52:2077–81.

2) Khaw KT, Dowsett M, Folkerd E, et al. Endogenous testosterone and mortality due to all causes, cardiovascular disease, and cancer in men: European prospective investigation into cancer in Norfolk (EPIC-Norfolk) Prospective Population Study. Circulation 2007;116:2694–

3) Shores MM, Matsumoto AM, Sloan KL, et al. Low serum testosterone and mortality in male veterans. Arch Intern Med 2006;166:1660–5.

4) Laughlin GA, Barrett-Connor E, Bergstrom J. Low serum testosterone and mortality in older men. J Clin Endocrinol Metab 2008;93:68–75.

5) Malkin, Chris J., et al. "Low serum testosterone and increased mortality in men with coronary heart disease." Heart (2010): hrt-2010.

6) Low Testosterone Linked to Heightened Risk of Early Death ScienceDaily (Oct. 21, 2010)

7) deleted

8) Ma, Ronald CW, and Peter CY Tong. "Testosterone levels and cardiovascular disease." (2010): hrt-2010.

9) deleted

10) Alexandersen P, Haarbo J, Byrjalsen I, et al. Natural androgens inhibit male atherosclerosis: a study in castrated, cholesterol-fed rabbits. Circ Res 1999;84:813–19.

11) Nathan, Lauren, et al. "Testosterone inhibits early atherogenesis by conversion to estradiol: critical role of aromatase." Proceedings of the National Academy of Sciences 98.6 (2001): 3589–3593.

12) Nettleship, Joanne E., et al. "Physiological testosterone replacement therapy attenuates fatty streak formation and improves high-density lipoprotein cholesterol in the Tfm mouse: an effect that is independent of the classic androgen receptor." Circulation 116.21 (2007): 2427–2434.

13) Bourghardt, Johan, et al. "Androgen receptor-dependent and independent atheroprotection by testosterone in male mice." Endocrinology 151.11 (2010): 5428–5437.

14) Mackman, Nigel, and Susan Smyth. "Cardiovascular disease in women." Arteriosclerosis, thrombosis, and vascular biology 29.3 (2009): 277–278.

15) Xing, Dongqi, et al. "Estrogen and mechanisms of vascular protection." Arteriosclerosis, thrombosis, and vascular biology 29.3 (2009): 289–295.

16) Kitamura, Tetsuhisa, et al. "Reduction in incidence and fatality of out-of-hospital cardiac arrest in females of the reproductive age." European heart journal 31.11 (2010): 1365–1372.

17) Grodstein, Francine, et al. "A prospective, observational study of postmenopausal hormone therapy and primary prevention of cardiovascular disease." Annals of internal medicine 133.12 (2000): 933–941.

18) Cignarella, Andrea, Mario Kratz, and Chiara Bolego. "Emerging role of estrogen in the control of cardiometabolic disease." Trends in pharmacological sciences 31.4 (2010): 183–189.

19) Kones, Richard. "Recent advances in the management of chronic stable angina II. Anti-ischemic therapy, options for refractory angina, risk factor reduction, and revascularization." Vascular health and risk management 6 (2010): 749.

20) Katritsis, Demosthenes G., and John PA Ioannidis. "Percutaneous coronary intervention versus conservative therapy in nonacute coronary artery disease: a meta-analysis." Circulation 111.22 (2005): 2906–2912.

21) Hueb, Whady, et al. "Five-year follow-up of the Medicine, Angioplasty, or Surgery Study (MASS II): a randomized controlled clinical trial of 3 therapeutic strategies for multivessel coronary artery disease." Circulation 115.9 (2007): 1082–1089.

22) Soran, Ozlem, Aarush Manchanda, and Stephan Schueler. "Percutaneous coronary intervention versus coronary artery bypass surgery in multivessel disease: a current perspective." Interactive cardiovascular and thoracic surgery 8.6 (2009): 666–671.

23) Miller-Kasprzak, Ewa, and Paweł P. Jagodziński. "Endothelial progenitor cells as a new agent contributing to vascular repair." Archivum immunologiae et therapiae experimentalis 55.4 (2007): 247.

24) Imanishi, Toshio, Takuzo Hano, and Ichiro Nishio. "Estrogen reduces endothelial progenitor cell senescence through augmentation of telomerase activity." Journal of hypertension 23.9 (2005): 1699–1706.

25) Foresta, C., et al. "Reduced number of circulating endothelial progenitor cells in hypogonadal men." The Journal of Clinical Endocrinology & Metabolism 91.11 (2006): 4599–4602.

26) Iwakura, Atsushi, et al. "Estradiol enhances recovery after myocardial infarction by augmenting incorporation of bone marrow–derived endothelial progenitor cells into sites of ischemia-induced neovascularization via endothelial nitric oxide synthase–mediated activation of matrix metalloproteinase-9." Circulation 113.12 (2006): 1605–1614.

27) Iwakura, Atsushi, et al. "Estrogen-mediated, endothelial nitric oxide synthase–dependent mobilization of bone marrow–derived endothelial progenitor cells contributes to reendothelialization after arterial injury." Circulation 108.25 (2003): 3115–3121.

28) Masuda, Haruchika, et al. "Estrogen-mediated endothelial progenitor cell biology and kinetics for physiological postnatal vasculogenesis." Circulation research 101.6 (2007): 598–606.

29) Bolego, Chiara, et al. "Selective estrogen receptor-α agonist provides widespread heart and vascular protection with enhanced endothelial progenitor cell mobilization in the absence of uterotrophic action." The FASEB Journal 24.7 (2010): 2262–2272.

30) Spyridopoulos, Ioakim, et al. "Caffeine enhances endothelial repair by an AMPK-dependent mechanism." Arteriosclerosis, thrombosis, and vascular biology 28.11 (2008): 1967–1974.

31) Vornehm, Nicholas D., et al. "Acute postischemic treatment with estrogen receptor-α agonist or estrogen receptor-β agonist improves myocardial recovery." Surgery 146.2 (2009): 145–154.

32) Sudhir, Krishnankutty, et al. "Premature coronary artery disease associated with a disruptive mutation in the estrogen receptor gene in a man." Circulation 96.10 (1997): 3774–3777.

33) Tak, Tahir T., et al. "Beneficial effects of enhanced external counterpulsation therapy in patients with angina pectoris and congestive heart failure." European Journal of Preventive Cardiology 21.1 (2014): S141.

34) Xu, Jia, et al. "GW27-e0597 Enhanced external counterpulsation promotes reendothelialization capacity of endothelial progenitor cells via activation of Tie2-dependent signaling pathway in stable angina patients." Journal of the American College of Cardiology 68.16 Supplement (2016): C23.

34) Raza, A., et al. "Enhanced External Counterpulsation Therapy: Past, Present, and Future." Cardiology in review 25.2 (2017): 59.

35) Tartaglia, Joseph, et al. "Patients that respond to enhanced external counterpulsation are at decreased risk for major adverse cardiac events and have increases in endothelial precursor stem cells." Journal of the American College of Cardiology 65.10 Supplement (2015): A1651.

A Major Dogma of Mainstream Medicine

A MAJOR DOGMA OF MAINSTREAM medicine is the unquestioned benefit of statin drugs for atherosclerotic heart disease. Statin drugs may have a justifiable use in certain segments of the population, namely middle-aged men with known heart disease. However, use of statin drugs is not justified for women, the elderly, or in the primary prevention setting. This is true because for these groups, there is no mortality benefit to outweigh statin's adverse effects.

Familial Hypercholesterolemia: Higher Risk of Heart Disease

What about a subgroup of the population with a genetic mutation called familial hypercholesterolemia, in which the serum cholesterol is markedly elevated because of a mutation in the LDL receptor? This is a common mutation affecting one in 500 people. (1)

Mainstream medicine says that this genetic trait, familial elevated cholesterol above 300, carries a higher risk for atherosclerotic heart disease and increased mortality at a young age. In the heterozygous condition, the risk of having a "coronary event" before age 60 is about 50% in men and 30% in women left untreated. (1) Surely, if statin drugs have any utility, it must be for this group of people with elevated cholesterol due to a genetic disease. Many will say the extraordinary benefit of statin drugs for the familial hypercholesterolemia patient is "proof" that cholesterol causes heart disease. Let us take a closer look at this argument.

Case Report: A Woman with Multiple Thyroid Nodules on Statin Drugs

Ann, a 61-year-old real estate agent, came to see me because of a number of tiny thyroid nodules that had been previously biopsied with an indeterminate result. Her doctors couldn't decide if the nodules were benign or malignant, so they recommended thyroid surgery with a total thyroidectomy, *"just to be sure."* Thinking this a bit hasty, Anne came for a second opinion. I explained to Anne multiple tiny thyroid nodules are quite common in the population and most likely of no clinical significance. The vast majority of thyroid nodules can be followed with serial ultrasound.

Statin Drug for High Cholesterol

In addition, Anne had been taking a statin drug for high cholesterol and had obvious adverse drug effects, including muscle weakness, muscle pain, and memory loss. Anne's lab panel showed a cholesterol of 240, which is perfectly normal. I do not use the lab range that has been influenced by the drug industry. My usual approach in this scenario is to suggest a coronary calcium scan to assess the amount of underlying arterial plaque and to answer the question, *"Does Anne need a statin drug?"* Anne's calcium score test result came back "zero" indicating no need for a statin drug to prevent heart disease, as there was nothing there to prevent.

One Year Later

One year later, Anne was relieved and happy to learn the follow-up ultrasound scan showed the thyroid nodules were smaller in size, indicating that Anne certainly did not need thyroid surgery. Also, at this same visit, a repeat cholesterol lab panel showed that Anne's cholesterol, off the statin drug, had gone up to 330. The cholesterol had previously been 241 while taking a statin drug.

My Cholesterol Has Always Been Elevated

I then asked Anne if her cholesterol had ever been elevated in the past, and she said yes, it has always been elevated in the 300s her whole life. Not only that, her parents both have high cholesterol (in the 300s), and her sisters and brother also have the same levels. After hearing this, in one of those "Aha" moments, I said to Anne, *"You must have familial hypercholesterolemia!"*

Statin Drugs for Familial Hypercholesterolemia (FHC)

This complicates the issue. Indeed, Anne's mainstream medical doctor has been giving Anne a statin drug to lower her cholesterol from 330 to 240. In spite of the "zero" calcium score, should Anne be taking a statin drug because of the familial hypercholesterolemia (FHC), a risk factor for heart disease?

Simon Broome Registry in UK

The answer comes from a 2008 study from the Simon Broome Familial Hyperlipidaemia Registry in the United Kingdom. (1,2) In this study, 3,400 patients with familial hypercholesterolemia (FHC) were recruited from 21 clinics in the UK and followed for 26 years (46,580 person-years). (1) What did the researchers find? Here is a quote from the study:

> *Familial hypercholesterolaemia is associated with a substantial excess mortality from coronary heart disease in young adults but may not be associated with a substantial excess mortality in older patients. (2)*

Mortality Depends on Age

The authors looked at data both before and after the availability of statin drugs.

> *Before statin drugs were available, mortality from coronary disease was increased nearly a hundred-fold in young adults with FHC aged 20–39 years, and increased about four-fold for patients aged 40–59 years, but in those surviving through middle age, risk was similar to the general population. (1)*

In other words, if a patient survives past 60 with no heart disease, then they are no longer at increased risk. They have the same risk as the general population. They went on to say:

Both before and after statins became widely available, there was no excess coronary mortality in patients aged >60 years without known coronary disease. Patients surviving into older age before statins became available were therefore likely to be a highly selected group at lower risk of coronary disease. (1)

A Highly Selected Group at Lower Risk of Coronary Disease

The Simon Broome Registry of FHC answers our question. (1,2) At age 61, Anne still has no history of heart disease, and indeed her calcium score of zero indicated no plaque and no heart disease. Therefore, Anne must be a member of a *"highly selected group at lower risk of coronary disease."*

If Anne's high cholesterol over a lifetime placed her at risk, surely, she would have developed some evidence of heart disease by now. The fact that her calcium score is zero means that Anne is at low risk for heart disease. For Anne, therefore, adding a statin drug to prevent heart disease is not necessary and ill-advised. Statin drugs carry significant adverse effects, including reduced memory and cognitive function, muscle pain, neuropathy, etc.

An Argument Against the Cholesterol Theory of Heart Disease

Think about it. Thousands of people with familial hypercholesterolemia have elevated cholesterol above 330–350 for their entire lives. These people reach the age of 60 years and never develop heart disease. This is one of the strongest arguments against the Cholesterol Theory of Heart Disease. If elevated serum cholesterol causes heart disease, then surely all of these people with cholesterol levels of 330 their entire lives should heave heart disease. The Simon Broome Registry says they don't.

Reduce Cholesterol Naturally

The Simon Broome Registry study was re-assuring. Anne felt comfortable avoiding the statin drugs and instead used dietary modification and supplements such as Bergamot, a citrus food supplement. (3,4)

A Major Argument for Statins in Familial Hypercholesterolemia

It has been argued that the introduction of statin drug treatment for young patients with familial hypercholesterolemia has resulted in significant reduction in heart attacks and reduced mortality in this younger age group. (1,2) One might even suggest this "proves" the cholesterol theory of heart disease.

Refuting the Cholesterol Theory for Familial Hypercholesterolemia

Dr. Luca Mascitelli, in a letter to the editor of *Angiology*, (14) refutes this argument with a number of observations regarding patients with familial hypercholesterolemia. (14)

- Incidence of cardiovascular disease is NOT associated with the absolute cholesterol level. Drugs that reduce the cholesterol to much lower levels had no benefit in reducing mortality. (15,16)
- Cardiovascular disease in this syndrome may be related to inborn errors of the coagulation system rather than high cholesterol levels. (9)(13)
- Polymorphism in the prothrombin gene has been found in this group and is strongly associated with increased cardiovascular risk.
- Benefits of statin drugs may be due to pleiotropic, anti-thrombotic effects, rather than any cholesterol-lowering effect.

Dr. Eric Sijbrands studied a family-tree pedigree of familial hypercholesterolemia over two centuries and makes a few striking observations (11)

- "Many untreated patients with familial hypercholesterolaemia (about 40%) reach a normal life span."
- "Standardized mortality ratio was normal in the 19th century and rose to a peak in the 1930s to 1960s."
- "The variation in mortality suggests an interaction between genetic and environmental factors." (11)

Early MI in Young Males: Testing Protocol

The testing protocol for thrombophilia genetic disorders includes:

- lipoprotein(a)
- homocysteine
- antiphospholipid antibodies
- plasminogen activator inhibitor-1
- factor V Leiden mutation
- prothrombin variant
- 5,10-methylenetetrahydrofolate reductase (MTHFR) C677T polymorphism. (48–54)

It's More Complicated

Clearly, familial hypercholesterolemia is more complicated than the simplified version presented by mainstream medicine, which blames cholesterol as the guilty party. If cholesterol alone were the cause of heart disease, why would we have significant numbers of patients (about 40%) with this syndrome surviving to old age without heart disease? Why was the mortality for these patients normal in the 19th century and yet elevated now? We await further research to answer these questions.

♦ ♦ ♦ ♦ ♦

♦ References for Chapter 25

1) Neil, Andrew, et al. "Reductions in all-cause, cancer, and coronary mortality in statin-treated patients with heterozygous familial hypercholesterolaemia: a prospective registry study." European heart journal 29.21 (2008): 2625–2633.

2) Simon Broome Register Group. "Risk of fatal coronary heart disease in familial hypercholesterolaemia." BMJ: British Medical Journal (1991): 893–896.

3) Petersen, Line Kirkeby, Kaare Christensen, and Jakob Kragstrup. "Lipid-lowering treatment to the end? A review of observational studies and RCTs on cholesterol and mortality in 80+-year olds." Age and ageing 39.6 (2010): 674–680.

4) Mollace, Vincenzo, et al. "Hypolipemic and hypoglycaemic activity of bergamot polyphenols: from animal models to human studies." Fitoterapia 82.3 (2011): 309–316.

5) Familial hypercholesterolaemia: summary of NICE guidance, BMJ 2008;337:a1095

6) The benefits of familial hypercholesterolaemia by Uffe Ravnskov BMJ Rapid Response 4 October 2008

7) Wierzbicki AS, Humphries SE, Minhas R; Guideline Development Group. Familial hypercholesterolaemia: summary of NICE guidance.BMJ 2008;337:a1095

8) Miettinen TA, Gylling H. Mortality and cholesterol metabolism in familial hypercholesterolemia. Long-term follow-up of 96 patients. Arteriosclerosis 1988;8:163–7.

9) Sugrue DD and others. Coronary artery disease and haemostatic variables in heterozygous familial hypercholesterolaemia. Br Heart J 1985;53:265–8.

10) Postiglione A, Nappi A, Brunetti A, Soricelli A, Rubba P, Gnasso A, et al. Relative protection from cerebral atherosclerosis of young patients with homozygous familial hypercholesterolemia. Atherosclerosis 1991;90:23–30.

11) Sijbrands EJ, Westendorp RG, Defesche JC, de Meier PH, Smelt AH, Kastelein JJ. Mortality over two centuries in large pedigree with familial hypercholesterolaemia: family tree mortality study. BMJ 2001;322:1019–23.

12) Ravnskov U. High cholesterol may protect against infections and atherosclerosis. QJM 2003;96:927–34.

13) Jansen, Angelique CM, et al. "Genetic determinants of cardiovascular disease risk in familial hypercholesterolemia." Arteriosclerosis, thrombosis, and vascular biology 25.7 (2005): 1475–1481.

14) Mascitelli, Luca, et al. "After the failure of ENHANCEd cholesterol lowering in familial hypercholesterolemia, SEAS of problems with ezetimibe." Angiology 60.1 (2009): 127–128.

15) Whayne TF Jr. Is there a problem with ezetimibe or just ENHANCEd hype? Angiology. 2008 Sep 15 [Epub ahead of print].

16) Pedone C, Carbonin P, Kastelein JJ, et al. ENHANCE Investigators. Simvastatin with or without ezetimibe in familial hypercholesterolemia. N Engl J Med. 2008;358: 1431–1443.

17) Jansen AC, van Aalst-Cohen ES, Tanck MW, et al. The contribution of classical risk factors to cardiovascular disease in familial hypercholesterolaemia: data in 2400 patients. J Intern Med. 2004;256:482–490.

18) de Sauvage Nolting PR, Defesche JC, Buirma RJ, Hutten BA, Lansberg PJ, Kastelein JJ. Prevalence and significance of cardiovascular risk factors in a large cohort of patients with familial hypercholesterolaemia. J Intern Med. 2003;253:161–168.

19) Sugrue DD, Trayner I, Thompson GR, et al. Coronary artery disease and haemostatic variables in heterozygous familial hypercholesterolaemia. Br Heart J. 1985;53: 265–268.

20–21) deleted

22) Holmes, Daniel T., et al. "Lipoprotein (a) is an independent risk factor for cardiovascular disease in heterozygous familial hypercholesterolemia." Clinical chemistry 51.11 (2005): 2067–2073.

23) Neil, H. A. W., et al. "Established and emerging coronary risk factors in patients with heterozygous familial hypercholesterolaemia." Heart 90.12 (2004): 1431–1437.

24) Humphries, S. E., et al. "Genetic causes of familial hypercholesterolaemia in patients in the UK: relation to plasma lipid levels and coronary heart disease risk." Journal of medical genetics 43.12 (2006): 943–949.

25) Neil, H. A. W., et al. "Non-coronary heart disease mortality and risk of fatal cancer in patients with treated heterozygous familial hypercholesterolaemia: a prospective registry study." Atherosclerosis 179.2 (2005): 293–297.

26) Sijbrands, Eric JG, et al. "Mortality over two centuries in large pedigree with familial hypercholesterolaemia: family tree mortality study Commentary: Role of other genes and environment should not be overlooked in monogenic disease." BMJ 322.7293 (2001): 1019–1023.

27) Versmissen, Jorie, et al. "Efficacy of statins in familial hypercholesterolaemia: a long term cohort study." Bmj 337 (2008): a2423.

38) Unit, Epidemiological Studies. "Efficacy and safety of cholesterol-lowering treatment: prospective meta-analysis of data from 90 056 participants in 14 randomised trials of statins." Lancet 366.9493 (2005): 1267–1278.

39) Mohrschladt, M. F., et al. "Cardiovascular disease and mortality in statin-treated patients with familial hypercholesterolemia." Atherosclerosis 172.2 (2004): 329–335.

40) Neefjes, Lisan A., et al. "CT coronary plaque burden in asymptomatic patients with familial hypercholesterolaemia." Heart (2011): hrt-2010.

41) Caballero, Paloma, et al. "Detection of subclinical atherosclerosis in familial hypercholesterolemia using non-invasive imaging modalities." Atherosclerosis 222.2 (2012): 468–472.

42) Neefjes, Lisan A., et al. "Accelerated subclinical coronary atherosclerosis in patients with familial hypercholesterolemia." Atherosclerosis 219.2 (2011): 721–727.

43) Miname, Marcio H., et al. "Evaluation of subclinical atherosclerosis by computed tomography coronary angiography and its association with risk factors in familial hypercholesterolemia." Atherosclerosis 213.2 (2010): 486–491.

44) Medel, David Viladés, et al. "Coronary computed tomographic angiographic findings in asymptomatic patients with heterozygous familial hypercholesterolemia and null allele low-density lipoprotein receptor mutations." American Journal of Cardiology 111.7 (2013): 955–961.

45) Williams, R. R., et al. "Evidence That Men With Familial Hypercholesterolemia Can Avoid Early Coronary Death; An Analysis of 77 Gene Carriers in Pour Utah Pedigrees." Journal of Cardiopulmonary Rehabilitation and Prevention 6.4 (1986): 148.

46) Ferrieres, J., et al. "Coronary artery disease in heterozygous familial hypercholesterolemia patients with the same LDL receptor gene mutation." Circulation 92.3 (1995): 290–295.

47) Neil, H. A. W., et al. "Mortality in treated heterozygous familial hypercholesterolaemia: implications for clinical management. Scientific Steering Committee on behalf of the Simon Broome Register Group." Atherosclerosis 142.1 (1999): 105–112.48)

48) Sofi, Francesco, et al. "Thrombophilic risk factors for symptomatic peripheral arterial disease." Journal of vascular surgery 41.2 (2005): 255–260.

49) Marcucci, Rossella, et al. "PAI-1 and homocysteine, but not lipoprotein (a) and thrombophilic polymorphisms, are independently associated with the occurrence of major adverse cardiac events after successful coronary stenting." Heart 92.3 (2006): 377–381.

50) Margaglione, Maurizio, et al. "The PAI-1 gene locus 4G/5G polymorphism is associated with a family history of coronary artery disease." Arteriosclerosis, thrombosis, and vascular biology 18.2 (1998): 152–156.

51) Mansur, Antonio P., et al. "The involvement of multiple thrombogenic and atherogenic markers in premature coronary artery disease." Clinics 68.12 (2013): 1502–1508.

52) Guney, A. I., et al. "Effects of ACE polymorphisms and other risk factors on the severity of coronary artery disease." Genet Mol Res 12.4 (2013): 6895–906.

53) Martínez-Quintana, Efrén, et al. "Prognostic value of ACE I/D, AT1R A1166C, PAI-I 4G/5G and GPIIIa a1/a2 polymorphisms in myocardial infarction." Cardiology journal 21.3 (2014): 229–237.

54) Fatini, C., et al. "Searching for a better assessment of the individual coronary risk profile. The role of angiotensin-converting enzyme, angiotensin II type 1 receptor and angiotensinogen gene polymorphisms." European heart journal 21.8 (2000): 633–638.

CHAPTER

26

Evolocumab: Are You Joking Me?

RALPH IS A 48-YEAR-OLD DIVORCE lawyer who arrives in my office with a history of familial hypercholesterolemia. Every lab panel since he was a kid showed a cholesterol level of 340. Other family members had the same genetic abnormality, and some even died of heart attack at an early age. About 6 months, ago Ralph switched to a new doctor who was alarmed by his high cholesterol, and started him on a statin drug, which reduced his LDL cholesterol down to 95. However, thinking this was insufficient, the new doctor added evolocumab, to drive the LDL cholesterol even lower.

FDA Approved in December 2017

Amgen's evolocumab (Repatha), FDA approved in 2017, requires an injection every 2 weeks. At $14,000 a year, it is the most expensive cholesterol drug on the market. A similar PCSK9 inhibitor drug, bococizumab, under development by Pfizer, was discontinued after a failed study. (7)

Lowest LDL in History of Medicine

After evolocumab was added to his statin drug, Ralph's labs showed an LDL cholesterol of 30, the lowest in the history of Western civilization in a human. I looked at Ralph and asked him if he was all right. *"Not exactly,"* he said. Ralph has trouble sleeping ever since starting the cholesterol-lowering drugs. He has been experiencing troublesome tingling and burning sensations on his arms at night while trying to sleep. In a nutshell, Ralph is miserable, and wants to know if he can safely stop the cholesterol medication.

"A Lifesaving Miracle Drug"

Many newspapers and cardiologists proclaim that evolocumab is a "lifesaving" miracle drug. (1)(27) Let us review the data table showing the number of lives saved in Dr. Marc Sabatine's FOURIER study. (2) In this study, 27,500 patients on statin drugs for atherosclerotic heart disease were randomized to either drug (evolocumab) or placebo. The drug reduced the LDL-cholesterol by 60%, from 90 to 30 mg/dl.

Cardiovascular Death: No Lives Saved

At the end of the 2.2 year study period there were 251 cardiovascular deaths in the drug group and only 240 in the placebo group. There were 11 more deaths in the drug-treated group. There were no lives saved.

Death from Any Cause: No Lives Saved

There were 444 deaths from any cause in the drug group and only 426 in the placebo group—eighteen more deaths in the drug-treated than in the placebo group. No lives saved.

A Lifesaving Drug that Actually Kills More People Than a Placebo?

Perhaps someone can explain to me how this can be called a "lifesaving" miracle drug, when in fact more people died in the drug group and no lives were actually saved?

The Miraculous Benefit of Intensive Lowering of LDL Cholesterol

If one is coldly objective about the data coming in, one might say the PCSK9 drug trials have actually falsified the cholesterol theory of heart disease. Here we have the lowest LDL cholesterol ever achieved in the history of medicine, yet no lives are saved. (20)

Wait Just A Minute, FOURIER Showed Reduction in MIs

The FOURIER study data did show 171 fewer myocardial infarctions in the PCSK9 evolocumab drug group. Isn't this a real benefit of the drug? Here is what Dr. Harumi Okuyama had to say about that. (56) The data is biased and faked:

> *The composite end point included measures that were less objective; hence, the accuracy of these measures as used across 49 different countries could have been biased, with the exception of mortality. For example, troponin level is known to be elevated after coronary angioplasty, leading to more frequent diagnosis of MI in the placebo group . . . We speculate that the reported data do not substantiate the conclusions made by the original authors, and we recommend against accepting their conclusions as an endorsement of PCSK9 inhibitors. (56)*

Heart Attacks Kill People, Don't They?

I think we are all in agreement with the statement: *"Heart attacks kill people."* You might ask, how many people? According to Dr. Viola Vaccarino in the *New England Journal* of Medicine from 1999, early mortality after myocardial infarction is 16.7 per cent in men and 11.5 per cent in women. (58) If we have two randomized groups and one group has more heart attacks, then this should translate into increased mortality for that group. This is just common sense. The FOURIER evolocumab drug study showed the opposite. The placebo group had 171 more heart attacks yet did not show increased mortality compared to the drug group. Exactly how an FDA committee can overlook this blatantly obvious contradiction is mind boggling.

Effect of Intensive Cholesterol Lowering on Calcium Score

We have made the case for annual calcium score progression as our most important tool in the management of coronary artery disease. Where is the calcium score data for the FOURIER evolocumab study? The study neglected to obtain annual calcium scores, so there is none.

Remember, statin cholesterol-lowering drugs were studied with annual calcium score by Dr. Paolo Raggi in 2004. His study showed that 41 of 500 patients on statins had heart attacks over 6 years in spite of cholesterol lowering. The feature that defined the heart attack group was a greater than 15% annual calcium score progression, not the cholesterol level, which was identical for both drug and placebo groups. If calcium scores are obtained in patients on evolocumab, would this duplicate Paolo Raggi's 2004 results? This would be a good topic for future study.

Non-Statin Cholesterol-Lowering Drugs Abandoned

Non-statin cholesterol-lowering drugs have not fared well in the past. Statin drugs have the advantage over these newer drugs because statins not only lower cholesterol, they also have pleomorphic (anti-inflammatory) effects that some would say provide the real benefit.

High hopes were raised for the non-statin CETP inhibitor drugs including Eli Lilly's Anacetrapib and Merc's evacetrapib. Both were highly effective for reducing LDL cholesterol, yet both failed to reduce the rate of cardio-vascular events in patients with high risk cardiovascular disease. Because of failed clinical trials, both drugs were abandoned and never brought to market. In retrospect, perhaps the newer non-statin PCSK9 inhibitor drugs should all share this same fate. (7) In my opinion, lack of mortality benefit should have prevented FDA approval of evolocumab, which was approved anyway, rais-ing the question of behind the scenes political influence. It is indeed a difficult thing to walk away from a 500-million-dollar investment.

Concern for Adverse Neurocognitive Effects

The FOURIER evolocumab study reported no adverse effects from inten-sive lipid-lowering. I find this difficult to believe in view of the FDA warning letter asking for a prospective study of neurocognitive adverse effects in the PCSK9 Inhibitor treated group. (29,30) "Adverse neurocognitive effect" is a polite way to say loss of ability to focus, think, and remember. In other words, drug-induced dementia.

Dr. Kristopher Swiger wrote the following in 2015 in *Drug Safety*.

On both theoretical and empirical grounds, concern for adverse neurocognitive effects currently extends to PCSK9 inhibitors. (31) These events included delirium, cognitive and attention disorders and disturbances, dementia, disturbances in thinking and perception, and mental impairment disorders. (32)

Adverse Psychiatric Reactions with Intensive Cholesterol Lowering

Lower cholesterol level is associated with a number of adverse psychiatric reactions, such as increased risk of suicidal and violent behavior, depression, aggression, and impulsivity. (35–37) Dr. Eriksen wrote in *Psychiatry Research* 2017, *"Low cholesterol is a risk marker for inpatient and post-discharge violence in acute psychiatry." (*39) People with low cholesterol are more likely to commit violent crimes. (41) Dr. Beatrice Golomb found that low cholesterol was associated with *"severe irritability homicidal impulses, threats to others, road rage, generation of fear in family members, and damage to property."* (42)

Dr. Michael Tatley writes about "Psychiatric adverse reactions with statins, fibrates and ezetimibe" in *Drug Safety* 2007:

The reactions mentioned . . . include depression, memory loss, confusion and aggressive reactions. . . . The observation that other lipid-lowering agents have similar adverse effects supports the hypothesis that decreased brain cell membrane cholesterol may be important in the aetiology of these psychiatric reactions. (43)

Dr. Repo-Tiihonen investigated *"associations between total cholesterol levels, violent and suicidal behavior, age of onset of the conduct disorder (CD) and the age of death among 250 Finnish male criminal offenders with ASPD (Antisocial Personality Disorder),"* finding lower cholesterol a prognostic marker for early unnatural death and violent crimes. (44)

We Cannot Ignore the Massive Data of Negative Impact

In 2016 *Drug Safety*, Drs. Cham, Koslik, and Golomb reported on *"Mood, Personality, and Behavior Changes During Treatment with Statins: A Case Series."* Adverse events related to cholesterol-lowering drugs included violent ideation, irritability, depression, and suicide. These problems resolved when the drug was stopped and recurred when the drug restarted. (45)

Dr. Alfonso Troisi says in Neuroscience & Biobehavioral Reviews 2009 that *"we cannot ignore the mass of data showing a negative impact of low cholesterol in some clinical populations or healthy subjects."* (38)

U-Shaped Curve Associates Low Cholesterol with Increased Mortality

The finding of increased mortality at low cholesterol levels is not surprising and has been known for decades. In the 1990s, accumulated data from multiple studies showed that low cholesterol is associated with increased mortality. (46–53) The cholesterol data chart reveals a U-shaped curve in cohort studies such as the J-Lit, HUNT-2, and MRFIT. (46–53) Both the left and right arms of the curve show increased mortality. Dr. Halfdan Petursson from Norway says (2012):

Regarding the association between total cholesterol and mortality, our results generally indicated U-shaped or inverse linear curves for total and CVD mortality. . . . Our results contradict the guidelines' well-established demarcation line (200 mg/dl) between "good"' and "too high" levels of cholesterol. They also contradict the popularized idea of a positive, linear relationship between cholesterol and fatal disease. Guideline-based advice regarding CVD prevention may thus be outdated and misleading, particularly regarding many women who have cholesterol levels in the range of (200–270 mg/dl) and are currently encouraged to take better care of their health. . . . recommendations regarding the "dangers" of cholesterol should be revised. This is especially true for women, for whom moderately elevated cholesterol (by current standards) may prove to be not only harmless but even beneficial. (48)

In *Circulation* 1992, Dr. Judith Walsh says:

There is an association between low blood cholesterol and noncardiovascular deaths in men and women. There is no association between high blood cholesterol and cardiovascular deaths in women. (51)

In 1993, Dr. David Jacobs speculated on the reason low cholesterol is associated with risk of non-atherosclerotic death. He writes:

Cholesterol affects the fluidity of cell membranes, membrane permeability, transmembrane exchange, signal transmission, and other cell properties. Cholesterol is a precursor for five major classes of steroid hormones. It affects gluconeogenesis and immune function; its transport forms, the lipoproteins, also serve as vehicles for fat-soluble vitamins, antioxidants, drugs, and toxins. Thus, cholesterol plays general, fundamental, and highly specific roles in the economy of the body. . . . Several authors have recently suggested caution in the pursuit of low Total Cholesterol, recommending against Total Cholesterol lowering in persons with Total Cholesterol less than 225 mg/dl." (50)

Review and Meta-Analysis of PCSK9 Drug Trials

In 2018, Dr. Alessandro Battaggia reviewed all the PCSK9 studies and said there was no benefit. Even in trials recruiting familial hypercholesterolemia patients, there is a "tendency to harm" (57):

No beneficial relationship was found between LDL-C lowering and cardiovascular events explored by meta-regression; instead, there was a trend toward harm. For any of the other outcomes there was no significant association between LDL-C lowering and risk. . . . .A separate meta-analysis of trials recruiting familial hypercholesterolemia patients have showed a tendency to harm for almost all outcomes. . . . Therefore, at the moment, the data available from randomized trials does not clearly support the use of these antibodies. (57)

Conclusion

The lack of mortality benefit reported in the FOURIER study, in spite of the lowest LDL levels in medical history is not surprising, since increased mortality associated with low cholesterol has been known for decades. In addition, it is clear from both failed CETP inhibitor drug trials and the PCSK9 drug trials that lowering cholesterol with a non-statin drug is a futile exercise that provides no health benefit. I would agree with Dr. Alessandro Battaggia's report that intensive cholesterol lowering has a *"tendency to harm."* (57) This is a medical practice that should be halted immediately.

♦ ♦ ♦ ♦ ♦

◆ References for Chapter 26

1) New wonder drug can 'slash the risk of heart attack, stroke or death by a QUARTER' compared with just statins. The Sun U.K.

2) Sabatine, Marc S., et al. "Evolocumab and clinical outcomes in patients with cardiovascular disease." New England Journal of Medicine 376.18 (2017): 1713–1722.

3) Correspondence. Evolocumab in Patients with Cardiovascular Disease August 24, 2017. N Engl J Med 2017; 377:785–788 Rita F. Redberg, M.D. University of California, San Francisco, San Francisco, CA

4) Mar 22, 2017 Forbes Magazine. Not All Cardiologists Trust Amgen's Cholesterol Drug Study John LaMattina, Contributor

5) Mascitelli, Luca, and Mark R. Goldstein. "Questioning the safety and benefits of evolocumab." The Lancet Diabetes & Endocrinology 6.1 (2018): 11.

6) Cholesterol lowering – proven or not? Repatha Malcolm Kendrick.

7) Pfizer Ends Development Of Its PCSK9 Inhibitor 'November 1, 2016 by Larry Husten CardioBrief

8) Is the drug industry honest? Uffe Ravsnskov MD

9) Does the New Cholesterol Drug Repatha Save Lives? Is evolocumab (Repatha) a breakthrough for treating high cholesterol? Or is it an expensive drug that won't save any lives? Joe Graedon March 27, 2017

10) Lustig, Robert H., and Aseem Malhotra. "The cholesterol and calorie hypotheses are both dead—it is time to focus on the real culprit: insulin resistance." Stroke 13 (2018): 57.

11) Dixon, Dave L., et al. "Clinical utility of evolocumab in the management of hyperlipidemia: patient selection and follow-up." Drug design, development and therapy 11 (2017): 2121.

12) ACCP CARDIOLOGY PRN JOURNAL CLUB NEWSLETTER March 2017 |Evolocumab and Clinical Outcomes in Patients with Cardiovascular Disease (FOURIER) Evolocumab and Clinical Outcomes in Patients with Cardiovascular Disease

13) Evolocumab for High Cholesterol New Evidence Update ICER Sep 11 2017

14) Will Evolocumab Help With Coronary Heart Disease? By Naveed Saleh, MD, MS | Reviewed by Richard N. Fogoros, MD Updated April 03, 2018

15) Amgen's FOURIER cardiovascular outcomes trial. While the landmark study proved Repatha's heart benefits, results showed the drug had no statistically significant effect on cardiovascular death.

16) Giugliano, Robert P., et al. "Clinical Efficacy and Safety of Evolocumab in High-Risk Patients Receiving a Statin: Secondary Analysis of Patients With Low LDL Cholesterol Levels and in Those Already Receiving a Maximal-Potency Statin in a Randomized Clinical Trial." JAMA cardiology 2.12 (2017): 1385–1391.

17) Mar 10, 2018 The ODYSSEY Trial Ends Well — But Will It Be Enough? Larry Husten, Contributor Forbes

18) Praluent Cuts Deaths by 29% for Those With Highest Cholesterol Levels, ODYSSEY Finds Mary Caffrey Coverage of the 67th Scientific Session of the American College of Cardiology.

19) Dark arts pushing heart drugs Jerome Burne | 20th March 2016

20) The new pretender by Bryan Hubbard May 2017 (Vol. 28 Issue 2)

21) How To Save Zero Lives For The Low, Low Cost Of Two Million Dollars And Change, Tom Naughton April 19, 2018

22) More cholesterol craziness 08/07/2017 DRUG BUST by Alan Cassels

23) Sick Pharma Commercial: Repatha – Pay or Die! Uncle Vince

24) deleted

25) New Cholesterol Drugs Protect High Risk Heart Patients: MORE FAKE NEWS! Mar 17 2017 David Brownstein MD

26) Bohula, Erin A., et al. "Inflammatory and cholesterol risk in the Fourier trial (further cardiovascular outcomes research with PCSK9 inhibition in patients with elevated risk)." Circulation (2018): CIRCULATIONAHA-118.

27) THE WALL STREET JOURNAL June 20 2017 Sumathi Reddy. A Cholesterol Drug Tug-of-War.

28) The ODYSSEY trial is first clinical trial to show a mortality benefit with a PCSK9 inhibitor—there was no such reduction observed in the FOURIER trial. TCTMD HeartBeat. ACC2018 By Michael O'Riordan March 10, 2018

29) This 'miracle drug' is really nothing but a dangerous dud. Health Sciences Institute 3/27/17.

30) FDA CENTER FOR DRUG EVALUATION AND RESEARCH APPLICATION NUMBER 125559Orig1s000 SUMMARY REVIEW

31) Swiger, Kristopher J., and Seth S. Martin. "PCSK9 Inhibitors and Neurocognitive Adverse Events: Exploring the FDA Directive and a Proposal for N-of-1 Trials." Drug Saf 38 (2015): 519–526.

32) Early Evidence Linking PCSK9 Inhibitors to Neurocognitive Adverse Events: Does Correlation Imply Causation? Jun 01, 2015 | Kristopher Swiger, MD; Seth Shay Martin, MD, MHS, FACC Expert Analysis

33) New cholesterol-lowering blockbusters fast track to dementia.Health Science Institute.

34) Praluent: New Cholesterol Drugs Get Riskier By The Day Editor | January 15, 2015

35) Kunugi, Hiroshi, et al. "Low serum cholesterol in suicide attempters." Biological Psychiatry 41.2 (1997): 196–200.

36) Vevera, J., et al. "Cholesterol concentrations in violent and non-violent women suicide attempters." European Psychiatry 18.1 (2003): 23–27.

37) Stevenson, R. J., and H. M. Francis. "The role of cholesterol in disorders of brain and behavior: human and animal perspectives." Handbook of cholesterol. Wageningen Academic Publishers, 2016. 291–298.

38) Troisi, Alfonso. "Cholesterol in coronary heart disease and psychiatric disorders: same or opposite effects on morbidity risk?." Neuroscience & Biobehavioral Reviews 33.2 (2009): 125–132.

39) Eriksen, Bjørn Magne S., et al. "Low cholesterol level as a risk marker of inpatient and post-discharge violence in acute psychiatry–A prospective study with a focus on gender differences." Psychiatry research 255 (2017): 1–7.

40) Banach, M., et al. "Intensive LDL-cholesterol lowering therapy and neurocognitive function." Pharmacology & therapeutics 170 (2017): 181.

41) Golomb, Beatrice A., Håkan Stattin, and Sarnoff Mednick. "Low cholesterol and violent crime." Journal of Psychiatric Research 34.4–5 (2000): 301–309.

42) Golomb, Beatrice A., T. Kane, and Joel E. Dimsdale. "Severe irritability associated with statin cholesterol-lowering drugs." Qjm 97.4 (2004): 229–235.

43) Tatley, Michael, and Ruth Savage. "Psychiatric adverse reactions with statins, fibrates and ezetimibe." Drug Safety 30.3 (2007): 195–201.

44) Repo-Tiihonen, E., et al. "Total serum cholesterol level, violent criminal offences, suicidal behavior, mortality and the appearance of conduct disorder in Finnish male criminal offenders with antisocial personality disorder." European archives of psychiatry and clinical neuroscience 252.1 (2002): 8.

45) Cham, Stephanie, Hayley J. Koslik, and Beatrice A. Golomb. "Mood, Personality, and Behavior Changes During Treatment with Statins: A Case Series." Drug safety-case reports 3.1 (2016): 1.

46) Nago N, Ishikawa S, Goto T, Kayaba K. Low cholesterol is associated with mortality from stroke, heart disease, and cancer: the Jichi Medical School Cohort Study. J Epidemiol 2011;21:67–74.

47) Jeong, Su-Min, et al. "Association of change in total cholesterol level with mortality: A population-based study." PloS one 13.4 (2018): e0196030.

48) Petursson, Halfdan, et al. "Is the use of cholesterol in mortality risk algorithms in clinical guidelines valid? Ten years prospective data from the Norwegian HUNT 2 study." (2011). Journal of evaluation in clinical practice 18.1 (2012): 159–168.

49) Matsuzaki, Masunori, et al. "Large Scale Cohort Study of the Relationship Between Serum Cholesterol Concentration and Coronary Events With Low-Dose Simvastatin Therapy in Japanese Patients With Hypercholesterolemia. Primary Prevention Cohort Study of the Japan Lipid Intervention Trial (J-LIT)." Circulation journal 66.12 (2002): 1087–1095

50) Jacobs Jr, David R. "Why is low blood cholesterol associated with risk of nonatherosclerotic disease death?." Annual review of public health 14.1 (1993): 95–114.

51) Hulley, Stephen B., Judith MB Walsh, and Thomas B. Newman. "Health policy on blood cholesterol. Time to change directions." Circulation 86.3 (1992): 1026–1029. Health policy on blood cholesterol Time to change directions Hulley Stephen Judith Walsh Circulation 1992

52) Muldoon, Matthew F., et al. "Low or lowered cholesterol and risk of death from suicide and trauma." Metabolism 42.9 (1993): 45–56.

53) Kaplan, Jay R., et al. "Assessing the observed relationship between low cholesterol and violence-related mortality." Annals of the New York Academy of Sciences 836.1 (1997): 57–80

54) Iso, Hiroyasu, et al. "Serum cholesterol levels and six-year mortality from stroke in 350,977 men screened for the multiple risk factor intervention trial." New England Journal of Medicine 320.14 (1989): 904–910.

55) Kim, Yong-Ku, et al. "Low serum cholesterol is correlated to suicidality in a Korean sample." Acta Psychiatrica Scandinavica 105.2 (2002): 141–148

56) Okuyama, Harumi, et al. "A Critical Review of the Consensus Statement from the European Atherosclerosis Society Consensus Panel 2017." Pharmacology 101.3–4 (2018): 184–218.

57) Battaggia, Alessandro, Andrea Scalisi, and Alberto Donzelli. "The systematic review of randomized controlled trials of PCSK9 antibodies challenges their "efficacy breakthrough" and "the lower, the better" theory." Current medical research and opinion just-accepted (2018): 1–12.

58) Vaccarino, Viola, et al. "Sex-based differences in early mortality after myocardial infarction." New England journal of medicine 341.4 (1999): 217–225.

Is Your Drug from the Medical Museum?

IF YOU ARE A CURIOUS tourist, you might visit the local Medical Museum, where you will be amused by the well-preserved jars of medical specimens and tissue samples. There you will also find relics of past medical treatments, such as jars of leeches and old machines, like the iron lung. Perhaps the drug your doctor prescribes for you belongs in the Medical Museum. In 2015, Dr. Donald J Miller, former chief of cardiac surgery at University of Washington Medical Center, says statin drugs belong in the Medical Museum:

> *In the future, medical historians may liken the prescribing of statins to lower blood cholesterol with the old medical practice of bloodletting (1)*

Statin Cholesterol Pill in the Medical Museum?

The cholesterol test and statin cholesterol pills were first relegated to the Medical Museum in 2004 with publication of the calcium score study by Paolo Raggi from Tulane University. Dr. Raggi recruited 500 patients with heart disease on statin drugs, followed for 6 years with annual calcium score and cholesterol. Of the 500 patients in the study, 41 suffered heart attacks. In this group, annual calcium score progression was greater than 15%. For the other 450 heart-attack-free patients, annual calcium score progression was less than 15%. Surprisingly, the serum cholesterol was the same for the two groups, those who had heart attacks and those who were heart-attack-free. Dr. Raggi's study was nothing less than a paradigm shift in the management of heart disease. The serum cholesterol test and statin drugs belong in the Medical Museum. The cholesterol test has been replaced by the annual calcium score. However, mainstream cardiology has ignored and buried the Raggi study for years.

There is good news for those of us with a high calcium score. If we can modify diet and life style to reduce calcium score progression to less than 15% per year, then we have the same excellent prognosis as our neighbors with low calcium scores, regardless of how high our starting calcium score number. According to Dr Raggi's 2004 study, those of us with high calcium score over 1,000 enjoy the same excellent prognosis as those with lower scores of 50-100 provided we succeed in reducing annual progression to under 15% per year.

Why is calcium score so much better than cholesterol testing? Think about it. The serum cholesterol is a measurement of a blood substance distant from the wall of the artery. The calcium score measures the disease progression in the wall of the artery, exactly where the disease is located.

What Is the Calcium Score Test?

The calcium score is a CAT scan (computerized axial tomography) without IV contrast (plain) limited to the heart with imaging of the coronary arteries. The computer adds up the calcium in the coronary arteries to yield a "calcium score" representing the amount of calcium in the coronary arteries. The calcium score correlates with future mortality from heart disease. The higher the calcium score, the higher the mortality.

How to Reduce Calcium Score?

Dr. Budoff studied aged garlic showing excellent result for reducing progression of calcium score. The women's health initiative study showed that the estrogen-treated arm of the study reduced calcium score by 35%.

What About Statin Drugs for Calcium Score?

Multiple placebo-controlled studies show statin drugs provide the same benefit as placebo for calcium score. Some studies actually show worsening calcium score with statin drugs. Statin drugs belong in the Medical Museum. Similarly, studies show no correlation between serum cholesterol and calcium score, falsifying the idea that cholesterol causes arterial calcification.

Summary

You are now at the end of this book. We have traveled a long road together, reviewing causes and treatments for coronary artery disease, including diet and lifestyle modification. We have reviewed the medical studies proving the cholesterol hypothesis to be false, and we have explored mainstream as well as alternate explanations for the etiology of atherosclerotic heart disease. Again, the idea that cholesterol is the sole cause of heart disease has been shown to be an oversimplification, superseded and replaced by the "Leaky Gut LPS Theory of Cardiovascular Disease, associated with low-level endotoxemia, obesity, metabolic syndrome, and diabetes. More recently, 16s Ribosome techniques revealed polymicrobial biofilm colonizing the atherosclerotic plaque.

The vascular tree is not an inert system of pipes. It is a colony of living cells with the ability to regenerate, working in harmony with the immune system, the autonomic nervous system, and all the organs in the body. The vascular tree is not static, it is alive, with the ability to vaso-constrict or vaso-dilate, as instructed by the autonomic nervous system. The atherosclerotic plaque in the coronary artery, although often compared with the sediment clogging our kitchen drain, is actually quite different, composed of living cells and biologic substances that ebb in and out of the arterial wall by various transport mechanisms. Unlike your kitchen drain pipe, which cannot regenerate collateral vessels, your coronary arteries can. These collateral vessels are equivalent to "nature's bypass" around an occluded artery. Perhaps this is why invasive procedures with the "plumbing approach" provide outcomes similar to medical treatment.

The good news is we now have the ability to image the calcium in the artery with CAT scans and to measure it with the calcium score test. This tool give us the most powerful means to evaluate heart-attack risk, and to monitor response to treatment. This is the paradigm shift that this book empowers you to embrace fully. There is hope. Atherosclerotic coronary artery disease can be stopped and reversed. This book shows you how to do just that.

Give a copy of this book to your friends, family members, and cardiologists. And, don't forget to sign up for my free newsletter at: http://www.jeffreydachmd.com.

Jeffrey Dach, MD

♦   ♦   ♦   ♦   ♦

♦ References for Chapter 27

1) Miller Jr, Donald W. "Fallacies in modern medicine: statins and the cholesterol-heart hypothesis." Journal of American Physicians and Surgeons 20.2 (2015): 54–57.

Made in the USA
Columbia, SC
28 August 2019